The BODYBLISS Protocol – Effortlessly Attain and Maintain Your Ideal Weight Forever

Copyright © 2020 Sara Palmer Hussey

First published 30th May 2020

This edition was published on 12th November 2021

All rights reserved.

No part of this book may be reproduced or transmitted in any form or by any means, electronic or mechanical, including photocopy, recording, or any information storage and retrieval system, without permission in writing from the author.

This book is dedicated to my father, Brian Hussey (1937-2003), a devoted biologist, whose fascination with the study of life inspired the awe and wonder with which I approach this field of science.

Contents

Introduction	7
Chapter One – Timing	16
Chapter Two – Mindset	54
Chapter Three – Nutrition	114
Chapter Four – Metabolism	159
Chapter Five – The Protocol	190
Conclusion	211
References	218

Introduction

Every year a new fad diet appears and we jump at the promise of losing our excess weight in record time for an important event or the arrival of summer. However, while occasionally successful, we often find that the weight loss turns out to be temporary and soon we are back where we started or even further away from our optimum weight.

What is optimum weight?
Optimum weight should be defined as our healthiest weight. It is not the weight dictated to us by the media, but instead it is the weight at which the body is healthy and strong and able to function at its most efficient level.

The World Health Organisation (WHO) determines healthy weight by our Body Mass Index (BMI), which is a number derived from our weight in kilograms divided by the square of our height in metres. So, for example,

> Optimum weight is not the weight dictated to us by the media, but instead it is the weight at which the body is healthy and strong and able to function at its most efficient level.

if you are 1.80m tall and weigh 80kg, your BMI is calculated by dividing 80 by 3.24 (1.8 x 1.8). In this example, your BMI would be 24.7.

So, what is considered a healthy BMI? The World Health Organisation classes only those with a BMI between 18 and 25 as healthy, those with a BMI over 25 are classed as overweight and those with a BMI over 30 are classed as obese. A BMI below 18 is considered underweight.

A growing problem
According to the WHO's 2016 statistics, there are more than 1.9 billion overweight adults in the world and, of those, 650 million are obese. 67.9% of the adult population in the USA and 63.7% in the UK fell into the overweight category and 36.2% and 27.8% respectively for USA and UK adult populations were classed as obese.

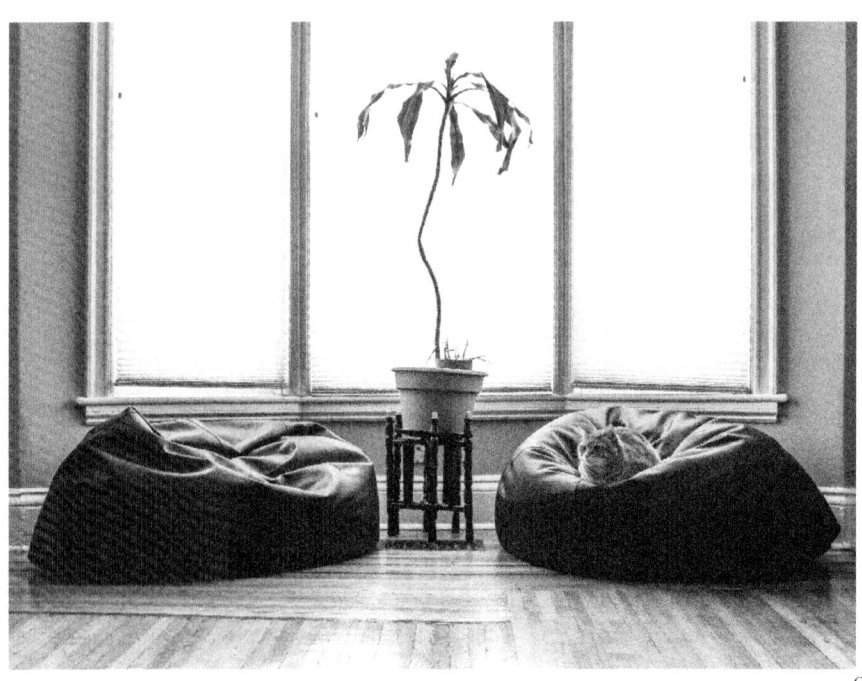

Between 1975 and 2016, the incidence of obesity has tripled and continues to grow at an alarming rate towards epidemic levels. In the UK alone, the National Health Service (NHS) spends over half a billion pounds per year for obesity-related issues.

Excess body weight is a health problem in itself and one that renders further health problems more likely, such as high blood pressure, heart disease, type 2 diabetes, respiratory problems, cancer and stroke. Excess weight also affects psychological wellbeing. In a society where thinness is equated with desirability, success and fitness, excess weight carries a psychological as well as a physical burden.

Is weight gain an inevitable phenomenon?
It seems that easy weight management is becoming more and more elusive. Why is there a trend towards obesity? Are we just naturally primed to gain weight?

Body fat and our ability to accumulate it have been prime factors in the course of our evolution as a species. We have a very high brain to body mass ratio compared to other animals (our brains make up 20-25% of resting energy requirements compared to 8-10% in other primates and 3-5% in other mammals, in infants under 10kg in weight, the brain accounts for over 60% of resting energy requirements). This high brain to body mass ratio necessitates the consumption of energy-dense foods. The evolution of the human brain is largely thanks to our ability to detect, assess and prioritise by taste preference the consumption of high-calorie foods.

Fat reserves: a survival mechanism
Survival was also ensured by our ability to accumulate and conserve body fat. Body fat acted as an energy buffer that could sustain daily energy requirements for several weeks without food and meant that we could survive ecological uncertainties, such as climate change, drought and famine.

Body fat, therefore, while also necessary for healthy growth, reproduction, immune and endocrine function, became a key survival factor.

> Hunger motivates us to hunt for food, while appetite is stimulated by the presence of food, so that we are more likely to eat than not eat given the urge and the opportunity. These mechanisms have secured our survival.

Consequently, the body is designed to take advantage of the presence of food to meet immediate energy requirements and add to fat reserves that can tide it over in moments of scarcity. Hunger motivates us to go out and hunt for food, while appetite is stimulated by the presence of food, so that we are more likely to be compelled to eat than not to eat given the urge and the opportunity. These mechanisms have secured our survival.

Our survival mechanisms are now working against us

However, in the modern, developed world, where access to food is ubiquitous, this survival advantage is starting to work against us, as escalating obesity rates testify. Food companies promote ever-larger portions of highly palatable, energy-dense foods that disrupt appetite regulation and drive overeating. They have also promoted the concept that it is acceptable and desirable to eat continually throughout the day: late at night, on the go, in our cars or on demand from the comfort of our armchairs.

Our survival instincts urge us to eat when food is available to cover us for potential future scarcity, but if food is constantly and consistently available without any balancing period of scarcity, the result is excess weight.

Unlimited access to food drives weight gain

In environments of limited accessibility or availability of food, obesity is rare. The so-called French paradox, which highlights French people's tendency to eat more fatty foods compared to the low-fat trend in the USA and other countries, while experiencing lower incidences of obesity and cardiovascular issues, may also be tied to limited access. The French traditionally tend to eat set meals together, 2 or 3 times a day, without snacks in between. Studies have pointed to the cardio-protective qualities of resveratrol in wine (the French have one of the highest wine consumption rates in the world) as the determining factor of this French paradox, but timing and access are almost certainly contributing factors, as well as the failure of low-fat diets, which we will cover later in this book.

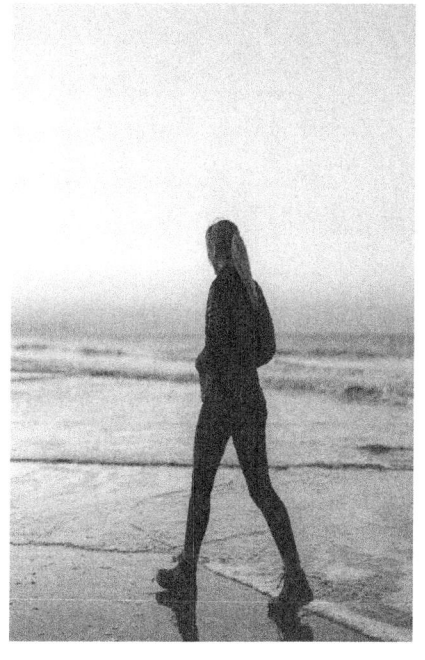

The body: friend or foe?

It can sometimes feel like we are waging war against our own bodies that do not get behind our goals. We want to lose weight and yet our bodies are urging us to eat more. Many diets arm us with a list of prohibited foods that our minds then demonically obsess over and drive us to eat. Our rational mind caves against the greater force of cravings and the subsequent feelings of failure can lead us to despair over ever achieving our goal of optimum weight.

All of which leads us to ask the question: Are there any friendly processes in the body that are on our side when it comes to successful weight management? Can we tap into any systems that actually facilitate weight management rather than falling victim to those that constantly thwart our efforts?

The answer is yes and this book will take you through a number of simple methods that support your body's ability to effortlessly attain and maintain your optimum weight.

> This book will take you through a number of simple methods that support your body's ability to effortlessly attain and maintain your optimum weight.

A comprehensive healthy approach
This book is focused on providing an effective and comprehensive protocol that not only achieves weight loss in the short term, but also, more importantly, provides an easy-to-follow framework for a healthier lifestylein the long term, in which optimum weight is maintained with the minimum thought and effort.

The BODYBLISS Protocol is a healthy, holistic approach that does not force down the number on the bathroom scales for a special event or the arrival of summer at the great expense of your health and balance. Instead, it takes a 360-degree perspective of all the factors involved in weight management and is targeted at optimising health and wellbeing as well as helping to easily shift to a new balance of stable weight management.

We all know that sustaining weight loss can often be more difficult than losing weight, which is why the aim of this book is to give you the tools that not only work for a brief period of time, but that will also give you a blueprint for the rest of your life. Best of all, it is easy and healthy; you will not be compromising your health or struggling against yourself, instead, you will be strengthening your health, supporting mental balance and experiencing new levels of wellbeing.

Your Personal Best
This book is not about reaching an unrealistic weight goal; it is really about healing your relationship with your body. It is about setting down your weapons of punishment, leaving aside restrictive diets and gruelling exercise routines and developing instead an attitude of care and appreciation for the marvel that is your body. In this book, you will learn the keys to optimum health and discover that when we take care of certain important factors and work in harmony with the body, the body responds by sustaining a healthy balance, which means high vitality, a strong immune system, an upbeat mood, good digestion, beautiful skin, hair and nails, and a healthy weight.

The goal is to rediscover your optimum weight. Your optimum weight is a personal, individualised weight for your physical structure that is its healthiest. Through application of The BODYBLISS Protocol, it is a weight that is effortless to attain and maintain. It is a weight that feels comfortable and liberating, and one that promotes maximum body confidence. It is the weight at which

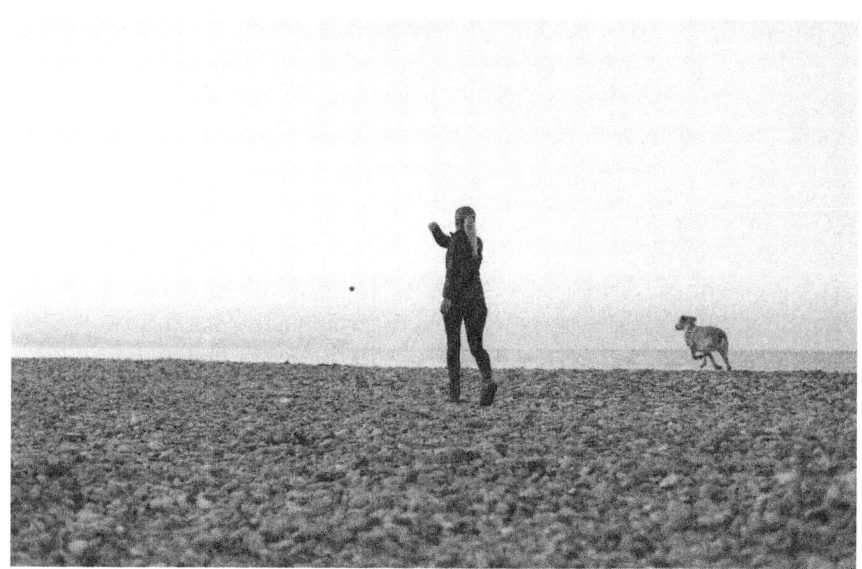

you feel free, healthy and at home in your body and you are no longer waging war against it, instead you are ensuring its best care.

What makes The BODYBLISS Protocol so different?
The BODYBLISS Protocol halts the war of hate against your body. It is a peace treaty, which paves the way for you to fall in love with your body again and learn to respect it and give it your best care. It is about being thankful for all the wonderful ways in which your body facilitates your experience of life and carries you through this journey. It is not about a specific body size or shape; it is about caring for your unique body, appreciating it and nurturing its best health.

> The BODYBLISS Protocol is a peace treaty, which paves the way for you to fall in love with your body and learn to respect it and give it your best care.

So, what is the key that The BODYBLISS Protocol has discovered that other diet books on the market have overlooked? Other diets and weight management systems have overlooked the key by searching for one, singular, headline-grabbing message. Where the body is concerned, no single process acts in isolation. It is unrealistic to believe that just one factor can be regulated to achieve the desired result when the determining factors are plural and interdependent. Regulating a single factor, for example diet, without taking into account the ramifications or the counterbalancing effects from all the interdependent systems involved, is simplistic, and the body is anything but simple.

By acknowledging the complexities of the human body, we will consider all the processes involved in weight management and we will address all the factors that can disrupt or support a weight loss goal. We will learn the importance of respecting our circadian rhythm and its influence on weight loss. We will also identify emotional factors that can trip us up and we will learn how to manage them. We will debunk some of the myths around diet and exercise and discover the power of the mind to influence weight and health generally.

Weight management is determined by multiple factors
The BODYBLISS Protocol is based on four pillars: timing, mindset, nutrition and metabolism. Our journey starts with timing and the body's circadian rhythm. Our circadian rhythm is the internal clock that regulates many different processes in the body. Knowledge of our circadian rhythm allows us to identify when to eat and when not to eat in order to optimise health and weight management. We will go on to deconstruct the energy equation, encompassing diet and exercise, that reduces weight management to the difference between calories consumed and calories spent, and we will find out how our mind can be our greatest enemy but also our greatest ally in our quest to lose weight.

Getting started
As you read The BODYBLISS Protocol, you can start applying as many tips as you like along the way. If you are someone who does not want to get bogged down in the science of why each factor is important, you can skip straight to the protocol section at the end of each chapter to put its steps straight into practice. Chapter Five pulls all four pillars of The BODYBLISS Protocol together into one plan of easy-to-follow steps that will lead you to your optimum weight. Whether you read this book word-for-word or jump around as if on a treasure hunt to find your favourite tips, by the end of this book, you should have a complete picture of all the factors involved in weight management, as well as a full tool kit of easy techniques in order to effortlessly attain and maintain not only your optimum weight, but also your best health, wellbeing and quality of life.

Enjoy the journey!

Chapter One – TIMING

We have learnt how, as a survival mechanism against periodic starvation, evolution has rendered our bodies more efficient at accumulating fat and less adapted to shedding excess weight. Therefore, we will need clever tools that short-circuit the body's resistance to utilising fat while also preventing the body from triggering the starvation mode, which safeguards fat reserves at all costs. In the following chapters, we will explore and learn to harness some straightforward strategies that render weight management easy. The first tool we will learn to master is timing.

For those of you who want to understand why this simple step is so effective at rebalancing your body and getting you on the right path towards attaining your weight goals, read on. For those of you less interested in the science and more interested in just getting the right tools and

> The timing of eating is of supreme importance in optimum weight management. In fact, the negative effects on weight of a bad diet can actually be mitigated by timing.

putting them into practice straight away, skip to "**TIMING PROTOCOL**" at the end of this chapter.

When you eat is as important as what you eat
In stark contrast to most other diets and weight loss systems, *The BODYBLISS Protocol* starts with a focus on ***when*** to eat as opposed to ***what*** to eat. Studies have shown that the timing of eating is of supreme importance in optimum weight management. In fact, research has shown that the negative effects on weight of a bad diet can actually be mitigated by timing.

> Research led by Dr. Satchidananda Panda at the Salk Institute, USA, has uncovered some interesting new revelations regarding the development of obesity and the timing of meals. In the past, weight gain and obesity have almost exclusively been attributed to excessive caloric intake. Dr. Panda and his colleagues set out to explore whether the timing of eating might be a decisive factor in weight gain too.
>
> Dr. Panda's research team put two groups of identical mice on an obesogenic diet (a diet designed to induce weight gain). Mice in the first group had unlimited access to food; they were allowed to eat at any time, as much and as frequently as they liked. Access to the same amount of food was restricted to an 8-hour window for the second group of mice.
>
> The results of the experiment were astounding. While the number of calories consumed by both groups was the same, the second group of mice appeared to be protected against the negative effects of their diet. Furthermore, they displayed several benefits from their new eating regime, notably improved motor coordination, increased thermogenesis and reduced serum cholesterol. As this and other research has concluded, timing (in particular, time-restricted feeding) offers an exciting strategy against weight gain and obesity.

So, why should the timing of meals offer such powerful protection against weight gain? What metabolic shifts are mitigating the normal effects of an obesogenic diet and how can we harness these to facilitate easy weight management? Let's take a deeper look at how respecting the body's cycles by timing our meals accordingly can facilitate easy weight management.

Ad Libitum Feeding
Ad libitum feeding refers to the free access to food enjoyed by the mice in the first group above that gained weight and eventually became obese. Ad libitum means as much and as often as desired. The mice in the first group had unlimited access to food and were allowed to eat at any time and as frequently as they liked. This very much represents our ability in modern society to eat whatever and whenever we like. There is a supermarket, a grocery store, a restaurant or a coffee bar on most streets, we can store large amounts of food in our homes and we can have all manner of foods delivered to our doorstep at all hours of the day and night.

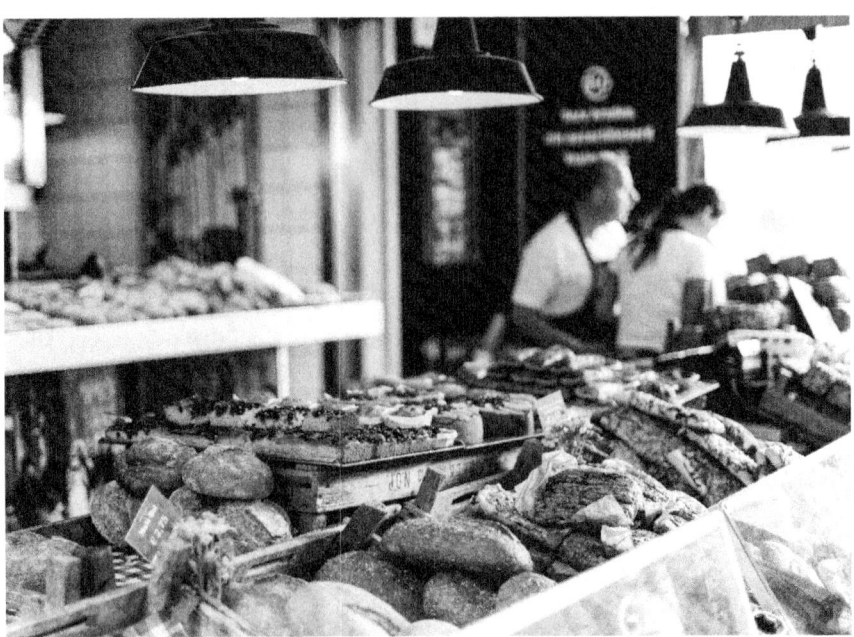

What happens in the body when we eat and why is timing so important? In particular, why is the break between one meal or snack and the next of vital importance in establishing whether the food will be added to our fat reserves or not?

Insulin
Insulin is a deciding factor between increasing or decreasing our fat reserves. Let's find out why.

Insulin is a peptide hormone produced by the glucose-sensitive β-cells in the islets of Langerhans of the pancreas. The glucose content of the food and drink we consume increases glucose levels in our blood and triggers the release of insulin into the bloodstream. Other components of our diet (such as the amino acids leucine, isoleucine, alanine and arginine) can also elicit an insulin response.

> Insulin is a deciding factor between increasing or decreasing our fat reserves.

Insulin's role is to keep blood glucose levels within a healthy range. Glucose levels in the blood go up after eating and the insulin released into the bloodstream will actively work to reduce the level back to normal by shuttling the excess glucose out of the bloodstream and into cells. Once blood glucose levels return to normal, the β-cells stop secreting insulin.

Most of the cells receiving their delivery of glucose, convert the glucose into energy, but fat cells and liver cells store it for future use. Liver cells convert the excess glucose into glycogen (via a process called glycogenesis) for short-term storage, or into fat (via a process called lipogenesis) to be stored in fat cells as a long-term reserve. Insulin's role in this process categorises insulin as an anabolic hormone, that is, it is a factor that promotes the building up of stored energy reserves as fat and glycogen.

When blood glucose levels fall (because we haven't eaten for a while or we have been exercising intensely and have used up the glucose in the blood to produce the energy required to sustain exercise), alpha cells in the pancreas will react by secreting a different hormone into the bloodstream that has the opposite effect to insulin. This hormone, called glucagon, mobilises stored energy reserves in order to increase blood glucose levels and keep them within a healthy range. This process categorises glucagon as a catabolic hormone, that is, it is a factor that promotes the reduction of stored energy reserves.

Therefore, glucagon has an opposite effect to insulin. Its goal is to raise blood glucose levels and it does so mainly by calling upon energy reserves stored in the liver (glycogen is broken down through glycogenolysis to supply glucose) and in fat cells (fats are broken down into fatty acids and glycerol through lipolysis, glycerol can be converted into glucose through gluconeogenesis).

Therefore, insulin and glucagon work together to maintain stable blood glucose levels. For the purposes of this book, it is vital to know that while insulin levels remain high, the body is not able to access and mobilise fat reserves and weight loss is difficult.

> While insulin levels remain high, the body is not able to access and mobilise fat reserves and weight loss is difficult.

Insulin Resistance

So, every time we eat, insulin is triggered and, while blood glucose levels remain high, insulin will be in the bloodstream doing its job of shuttling excess glucose into cells for utilisation or storage. Therefore, in the presence of insulin, the body tends to build up its back-up fuel reserves, for example as fat, and does not reduce its fat reserves.

This is not good news for the modern-day diet, which includes three main meals and various snacks, running from the moment we wake up to the moment we go to bed. Consequently, we only really clear the bloodstream of insulin and trigger the catabolic hormone glucagon when we are asleep. Remember, glucagon is the hormone that triggers the breaking down of our fat reserves for energy. Its action is essential for weight loss.

Our modern-day diet of frequent meals and snacks generates another compounding factor: insulin resistance. Insulin resistance is the process by which cells become increasingly insensitive to the action of insulin. It is a common issue, especially as we age, and is attributed to overstimulation. Overstimulation occurs when insulin levels remain high in the blood as a response to high blood glucose levels from a combination of overeating, continual snacking and a sedentary lifestyle.

> Glucagon is the hormone that breaks down our fat reserves. Its action is essential for weight loss.

In reaction to a bombardment of insulin, cells become progressively less sensitive to the action of insulin and, therefore, less able to draw in glucose from the blood for cellular energy production. This means that not only do energy levels fall, but also blood glucose levels remain high, which activates the additional release of insulin, and in turn worsens the insulin resistance of cells. When insulin fails to lower blood glucose levels, eventually type 2 diabetes develops.

Insulin resistance increases biomarkers of systemic inflammation, such as the pro-inflammatory cytokines, C-reactive protein, interleukin 6 and tumour necrosis factor-alpha (TNFα). It is also thought that increased levels of TNFα exacerbate whole-body insulin resistance in a self-perpetuating cycle. Chronic inflammation increases the risk of hypertension and diabetes, as well as being a precursor to many other diseases.

Insulin resistance in liver cells enhances the expression of genes associated with gluconeogenesis (the production of glucose from non-carbohydrate substrates, such as glycerol, alanine and glutamine), which further fuels high blood glucose levels and further exacerbates insulin resistance.

Fat cells and liver cells tend to retain their insulin sensitivity better than other cells, so insulin resistance in other cells increases the amount of glucose being converted into fat for storage, which accelerates weight gain. The continual activation of insulin through high blood glucose levels caused by continual over-eating and low energy expenditure, further fuels this vicious cycle that is a sure recipe for obesity.

> Insulin resistance increases the amount of glucose being converted into fat for storage, which accelerates weight gain.

How do we break this accelerating downward spiral?

Insulin Clearing
While the action of insulin is crucial to the stability of blood glucose levels, over-activation can unleash a downward spiral into obesity. Therefore, we need to be mindful about how many times a day we are triggering the release of insulin.

The only way to start to reverse insulin resistance is to clear the high blood glucose levels that are keeping insulin levels high. Allowing sufficient time to pass between one meal and another and increasing the time between the last meal of the day and breakfast the following day, are two ways to start clearing insulin daily and reducing the frequency of insulin release during the feeding window. Physical exercise accelerates insulin clearing and triggers glucagon.

Dietary improvements that are helpful in counteracting insulin resistance include increasing our intake of fibre, which slows down the absorption of glucose from a meal, increasing our intake of omega-3 fatty acids, which improve cell membrane fluidity and insulin receptor sensitivity, and ensuring we are integrating adequate levels of vitamin D.

To summarise, we have learnt that high blood glucose levels coupled with high levels of insulin increase fat storage, simultaneously preventing fat reduction. Therefore, in order to access fat reserves and start to shed unwanted weight, insulin needs to be cleared, not permanently (insulin has important benefits that we will learn about later), but regularly enough for the body to have the opportunity to switch to fat as a fuel source instead of just running on glucose.

> In order to access fat reserves and start to lose unwanted weight, insulin needs to be cleared regularly enough for the body to have the opportunity to switch to fat as a fuel source instead of glucose.

The only way to allow the body to start accessing and reducing its fat reserves is to bring blood glucose levels down low enough so that the body will temporarily cease producing insulin. Blood glucose levels will eventually fall if we stop adding to them with additional snacks, meals or glucose-rich drinks, or if we exercise.

When blood glucose levels fall, insulin release will halt and glucagon will be released to mobilise an alternative source of glucose to keep blood glucose levels stable. As we saw previously, this alternative source of glucose will be mobilised from the liver and from fat cells.

In other words, when we stop continually eating and triggering insulin release, the body will switch to an alternative fuel source, namely glycogen and fat. When that happens, we have tipped the balance in favour of weight loss. The body is then accessing and using its own existing fuel reserves to supply energy requirements. As fat reserves are mobilised for energy production, fat mass decreases and weight loss follows.

Time-Restricted Feeding
Let's go back to the mice and, in particular, the second group of mice that were protected against the weight gain experienced by the first group simply by virtue of a smaller feeding window. You will remember that the amount and type of food both groups ate was the same, but the second group of mice only had an 8-hour period of access to it.

Simply by limiting the mice's access to food to an 8-hour window, the second group of mice experienced none of the issues the first group of mice experienced and actually enjoyed benefits beyond weight management.

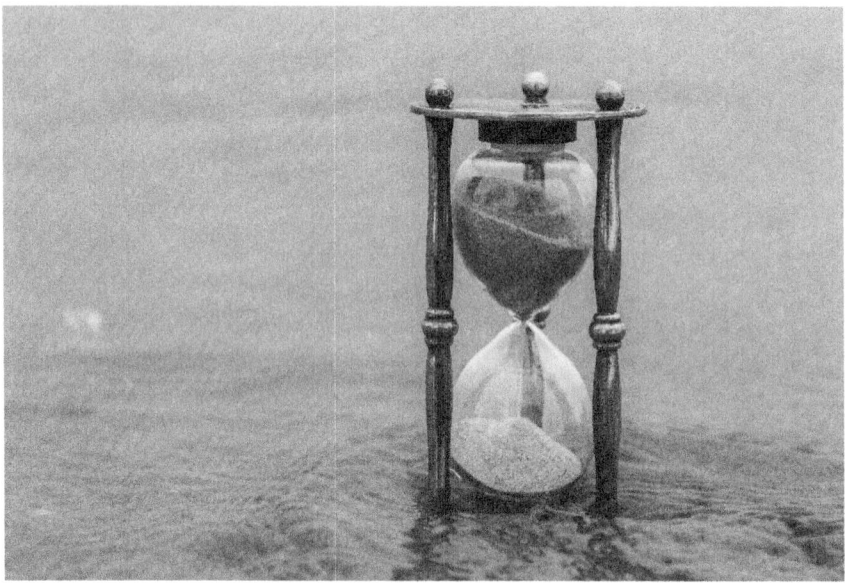

In further studies, the application of a larger 12-hour feeding window delivered the following benefits:

- Reductions in fat reserves despite obesogenic diet;
- Improvements in glucose tolerance and insulin sensitivity;

- Reductions in inflammation;
- Improvements in lipid profile;
- Favourable changes in gene expression;
- Increased production of ketone bodies;
- Protection from hepatic steatosis (fatty liver);
- Improved sleep;
- Improved heart rate variability.

In studies in which the feeding window was reduced to 8 hours, further benefits accrued, including:
- Improved aerobic endurance;
- Increases in lean muscle mass;
- Increased mitochondrial* biogenesis;
- Increases in mitochondrial volume, especially in the liver and brown fat;
- Decreased mitochondrial damage.

- mitochondria are the organelles inside cells in which energy is generated

This reduction of the feeding window to eight hours also reduced stomach distension, ghrelin (a hunger signal) levels and, consequently, appetite.

Therefore, even the simple technique of reducing our feeding window to 12 hours offers multiple benefits without any other lifestyle modification. Reducing the feeding window further and combining with a healthy diet, daily exercise, stress reduction and a regular sleep cycle, is a very effective regime for optimum health and easy weight management.

> The simple technique of reducing our feeding window to 12 hours offers multiple benefits without any other lifestyle modification.

By restricting food intake to a limited window of time, the body is no longer able to rely solely on glucose metabolism for energy. During the period of twelve hours or more in which there is no feeding, the body must mobilise alternative fuel sources from the liver and fat cells. This regular metabolic shift is beneficial not only for weight management but for health generally.

It has been hypothesised that forcing cells into oxidative phosphorylation (energy generation in the mitochondria in the presence of oxygen) could also be a valid therapy for cancer. Cancer relies heavily for survival and proliferation on glycolytic metabolic pathways (energy generation from glucose in the absence of oxygen). It has been shown that the increased mitochondrial activation induced during the fasting cycle, once glucose and glycogen have been depleted, promotes cancer cell death possibly by increasing levels of reactive oxygen species (ROS). This is known as the Warburg effect after the Nobel prize-winning scientist Otto Heinrich Warburg.

The Feeding/Fasting Cycle
The period of time in which no food is consumed is known as the fasting cycle. It is the time between eating your last morsel of food of the day and breakfast the following morning. Fasting physiology, which is triggered in the absence of feeding once stored energy starts being utilised, is a boon not only to weight management, but also to health and longevity. Much research is being carried out on this metabolic switch, that is, the point at which glucose and glycogen stores are depleted and fatty acids are mobilised. Depending on levels of physical activity, this switch can take place 6-8 hours after eating if the individual exercises or over 12 hours after eating if the individual is sedentary.

Therefore, in order to benefit fully from fasting physiology, we must have a fasting window of at least twelve hours. This corresponds to nature's day/night cycle and links us to the natural rhythms of the Earth.

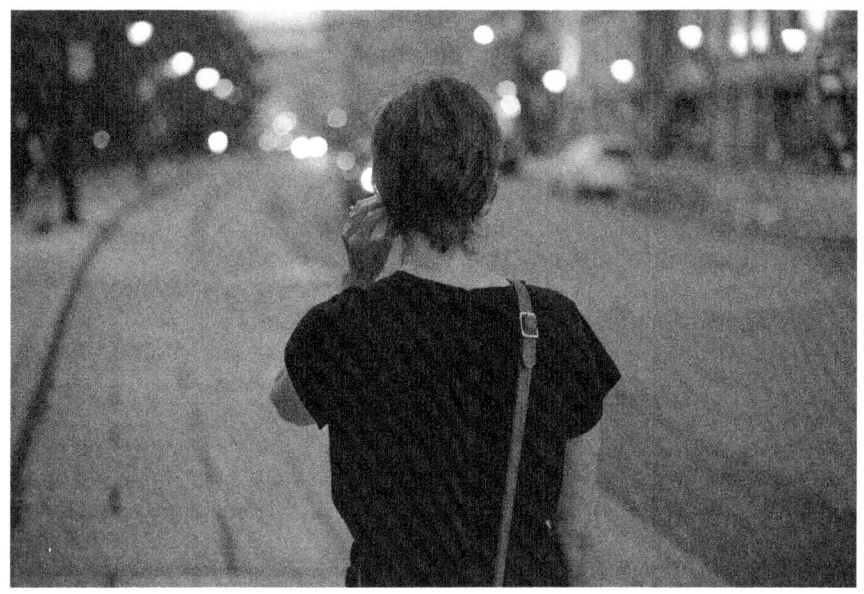

Our physiology evolved to adapt to daily cycles of nutrient availability, as well as the day/night cycle, in such a way that genomic programs are driven by these cycles. Coordinated oscillations at the transcript level allow for alternating cellular processes. Studies show that if these cycles are disrupted or if polymorphisms exist in clock genes, then insomnia, obesity, diabetes, depression and other health issues become more common.

During the fasting phase, the following processes occur:
1. Glucose levels fall;
2. Glycogen is depleted;
3. Insulin levels fall, facilitating lipolysis (breakdown of fat reserves);
4. Human growth hormone (HGH) levels rise, further facilitating lipolysis;
5. Autophagy (the removal or recycling of cellular debris) increases;
6. Cellular repair increases;
7. Oxidative stress decreases;

8. Inflammation decreases;
9. Triglycerides and LDL cholesterol levels fall;
10. Blood pressure falls;
11. AMP-Activated Protein Kinase (AMPK), which stimulates energy production, fat metabolism and plays a role in insulin signalling, increases;
12. NAD levels rise (NAD is a key player in energy production);
13. Ketogenesis increases, through increased fat metabolism, which further promotes protein deacetylation and autophagy;
14. Gene expression in genes related to longevity and disease protection increases;
15. Basal metabolic rate (BMR) increases;
16. Appetite control improves – ghrelin and leptin levels balance out;
17. Insulin resistance decreases;
18. Levels of brain-derived neurotrophic factor (BDNF), neurogenesis and neuro-plasticity increase;
19. Mitochondrial biogenesis increases;
20. Stem cell activation increases.

We can agree that the above list is pretty impressive and highly desirable on our quest for optimum health and effortless weight management. The fasting window is, therefore, a vital daily phase in order to promote better health and weight management. If eating is limited within the daylight circadian phase of 12 hours, weight management becomes effortless; so much easier than it is via caloric restriction, which can negatively affect our basal metabolic rate (BMR) and

> The fasting window is a vital daily phase for better health and weight management. Time-restricted feeding is easier than caloric restriction, which can negatively affect our basal metabolic rate (BMR) and erode lean muscle mass, whereas time-restricted feeding protects both BMR and lean muscle mass.

erode lean muscle mass, whereas time-restricted feeding (TRF) protects both BMR and lean muscle mass.

Furthermore, studies have shown that TRF, as well as intermittent fasting (IF), which involves eating less every other day, has the same effect as caloric restriction on healthy lifespan. In one study, rats fed every other day lived 83% longer than rats that ate every day.

TRF and IF have been shown not to slow down our metabolic rate or compromise nutrition, hormonal health or lean muscle mass in the way that caloric restriction does. The fatty acid-derived ketones the body produces during TRF and IF serve to preserve muscle mass and function. Nevertheless, a caloric deficit does unintentionally occur (subjects on TRF tend to naturally and effortlessly reduce total caloric intake by about 20% just by restricting their feeding window rather than by counting calories), and the decrease in calories is not interpreted by the body in the same way. Typically, subjects on TRF do not experience the same energy-saving effects as those common with caloric restriction, in which lethargy is an immediate consequence of a reduced BMR and hunger is triggered by increased hunger hormones, rendering caloric restriction a difficult regime to sustain. It becomes more and more of a struggle to resist the desire to eat beyond the very limited menu plans of such diets as hunger signals increase.

Both IF and TRF have a strong regulatory effect on blood glucose and insulin levels, reducing insulin resistance, glucose intolerance and type 2 diabetes. Oxidative stress is also minimised. Both IF and TRF upgrade important repair processes, such as the enhanced waste removal of autophagy, that take place during the fasting phase and mitigate damage and possible mutations.

TRF improves sleep and improves the function and impact on health of the glymphatic system. The fasting phase stimulates the glymphatic system during sleep, which clears out interstitial metabolic waste products from the Central Nervous System (CNS),

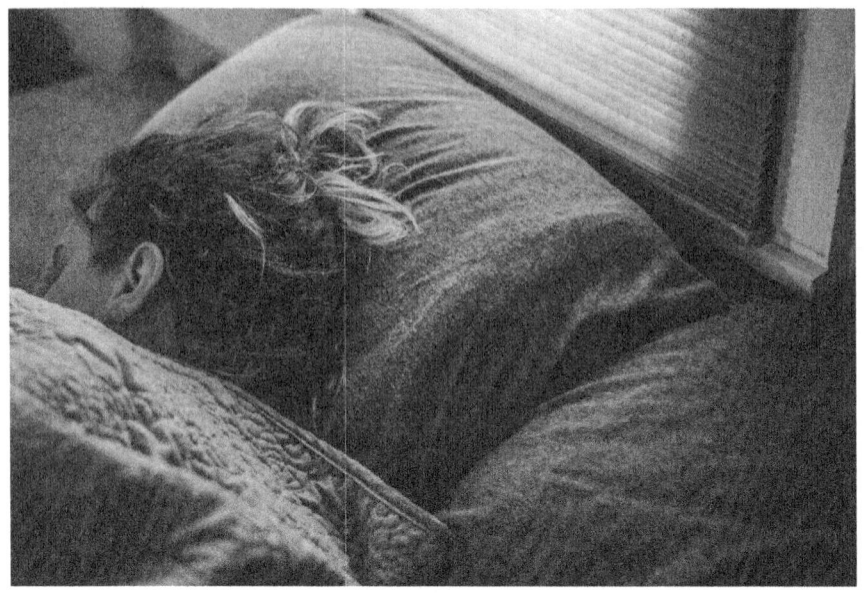

such as toxins and amyloid beta produced by neural activity in the brain during the day. This can have a protective role against neurodegenerative diseases, such as Alzheimer's and Parkinson's.

More prolonged fasting of over 48 hours increases the above benefits and also stimulates apoptosis, a process that clears out mutated or senescent (old, degenerating and pro-inflammatory) cells. Prolonged fasts are much harder to do, but can be done once or twice a year as a deep cleanse. Meanwhile, TRF provides an easy way to ensure daily autophagy, which should be enough to clear out protein aggregates and other harmful debris, while stimulating daily repair of the on-going damage caused by ROS (reactive oxygen species) and RNS (reactive nitrogen species).

Once we stop eating, it takes over 6 hours, depending on our BMR and activity levels, to deplete glycogen reserves and switch to fat oxidation. Ketone bodies, produced by fat metabolism, beta-hydroxybutyrate in particular, act as signalling molecules that alter gene expression by inhibiting class 1 histone deacetylases. They increase transcription factor PGC-1 alpha, which increases mitochondrial biogenesis and improves endurance and lean muscle mass. The quality of muscle mass is also improved by increased protein turnover. NAD levels rise and activate the SIRT1 pathway, which stimulates autophagy.

These benefits are optimised when the fasting phase is prolonged to 15 or 16 hours and the diet within the feeding window is healthy and balanced. Ideally, within the feeding window, we would eat just two or a maximum of three meals. Every time we eat, we know that the body secretes insulin that shifts the body into an anabolic, fat-storing state for the following hours. Therefore, in terms of weight management, it is best to trigger the insulin response only a few times a day and not by the constant snacking to which we have become accustomed.

Restricting the feeding window not only allows for insulin clearing and the metabolic shift to fat utilisation for energy production, it also highlights the numerous health benefits that can be enjoyed by respecting the body's circadian rhythm.

> Restricting the feeding window not only allows for insulin clearing and the metabolic shift to fat utilisation for energy production, it also highlights the numerous health benefits that can be enjoyed by respecting the body's circadian rhythm.

Circadian Rhythm

Life has evolved on planet earth under a consistent day/night cycle, which sets corresponding biorhythms in the body to optimally adapt internal processes to the environment. This physiological synchronisation between biological processes and environmental cues is known as entrainment. Through this rhythmic entrainment, our body has been primed to be active during the day and then to switch to a rest and repair mode during the night.

Most life on Earth displays biological processes that follow an endogenous (internally-regulated) rhythm of around 24 hours. This rhythm is based on an internal biological clock, but is also entrained by environmental cues, such as light and temperature, that is, reset, synchronised or adjusted by these external cues as occurs when we travel across time zones. Jet lag, for example, denotes the time it

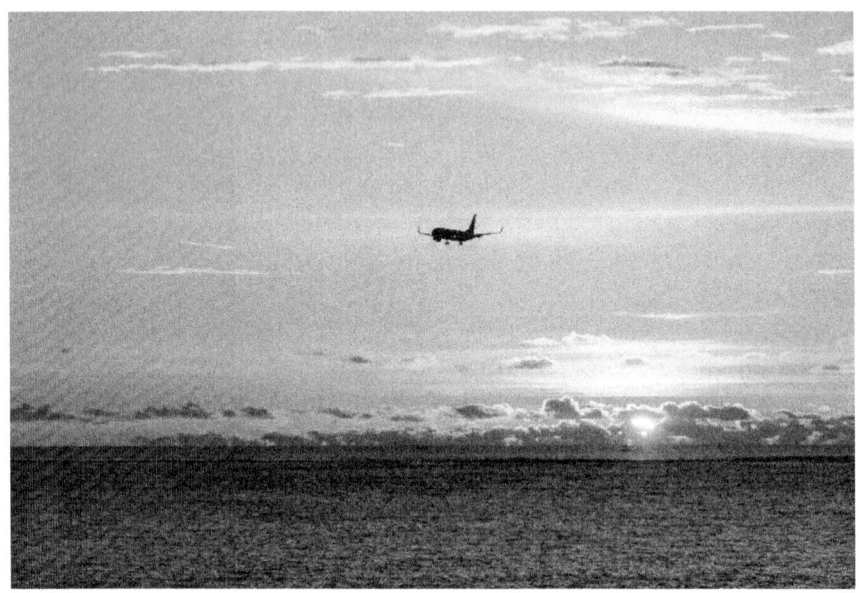

takes the body to readjust its circadian rhythm to fall into sync with the new environmental cues.

It has been shown that the success of transplants and other medical treatments may be increased through added consideration of the body's circadian rhythm. Also, with regards to pharmaceuticals, there is often a strong circadian regulation of the target of a particular drug, often a certain protein expression that the pharmaceutical drug seeks to inhibit. Therefore, if the expression does not become active until the evening, but the drug is taken in the morning, it will have no effect or will require an increasingly heavy dose before it has an effect, which also increases the side effects. If, however, the drug can be timed to match the peak expression of the target, then less of the drug will be required to maximise efficacy, while reducing potential side effects associated with the drug. This field of study is called chronotherapeutics and aims to reduce adverse reactions to medical interventions as well as increasing their efficacy.

We evolved to be diurnal creatures, that is, we are at our most active during daylight hours, hunting for food and eating, while we are equipped to store this energy intake to cover the rest of the day and night when we are not eating. During the time after feeding is complete, the body is able to digest and assimilate the food, use and store nutrients and efficiently eliminate waste. When we interfere with this cycle, each step of which requires time, we are interrupting vital processes that fall out of sync with the rhythm and flow of the body's circadian cycle. A disruption of the cycle of one process, has a knock-on effect on all interdependent processes, thus knocking the body's entire functioning off-kilter. Optimum health and easy weight management depend upon the synchronised rhythm and balance of all processes.

When our circadian rhythm is balanced between a distinct biological day and a biological night, the body is able to optimally assign activities to one mode or the other. Brain wave activity, immune function, hormonal production, autophagy, metabolic processes and cell regeneration all oscillate according to the distinct day and night modes of the circadian rhythm. For example, cellular repair, rest, brain development and memory processing are best suited to the night-time mode, while mental alertness, digestion, immune resilience and glucose availability are most needed during the day. A vital function of circadian oscillations in the body is to provide the crucial repair time required to mend the daily damage caused just from being alive, active and breathing.

Chronic disruption of the body's circadian rhythm can lead to insomnia, metabolic syndrome, obesity and decreased life expectancy. Studies have shown that mutations or deletions in the clock genes of mice result in erratic sleep patterns and hyperphagia (excessive appetite that drives over-eating) and obesity. Their metabolism is altered to favour glucose over lipid utilisation and they are predisposed to diabetes.

> Chronic disruption of the body's circadian rhythm can lead to insomnia, metabolic syndrome, obesity and decreased life expectancy.

Suprachiasmatic Nucleus
The body's primary internal biological clock is located in the brain, in a tiny region of the hypothalamus called the suprachiasmatic nucleus (SCN). Light information is projected directly along the retino-hypothalamic tract from photosensitive ganglion cells in the eyes to the SCN, which sends out signals to synchronise clocks in the rest of the body. These independent clocks, or peripheral oscillators, respond to a number of inputs, including light, exercise and feeding, but are all entrained or reset by the SCN.

The SCN interprets information from the eyes about day length and relays it to the pineal gland. The pineal gland regulates body temperature and produces melatonin, a hormone that regulates the sleep-wake cycle. The arrival of daylight triggers a signal from the SCN to the pineal gland to suppress melatonin secretion, and the body awakens. The arrival of darkness, on the other hand, activates melatonin secretion and induces sleep.

The SCN also influences the renin-angiotensin system and the hypothalamic-pituitary-adrenal axis with the activation of cortisol, adrenaline and noradrenaline. Studies have also shown neurological connections between the SCN and the heart, kidneys, adrenal cortex, liver, pancreas, spleen and white and brown adipose tissue.

The biological markers that track circadian rhythm are:
1. Body temperature, which reaches its daily minimum between the middle of sleep and waking;
2. Melatonin secretion by the pineal gland, which starts with the dimming of the light and surges prior to sleep;
3. Cortisol levels, which peak in the morning and fall to their lowest levels during sleep;
4. Heart rate, which reaches its daily minimum during sleep and its maximum shortly after waking.

Melatonin
As previously mentioned, melatonin is a hormone secreted by the pineal gland in the evening to regulate sleeping patterns. It is also an antioxidant that protects nuclear and mitochondrial DNA against oxidative stress. Moreover, melatonin improves the effectiveness of other antioxidants and, in contrast to antioxidant vitamins, such as vitamins C and E, melatonin's metabolites are also free radical scavengers. We can supplement our melatonin levels by eating foods

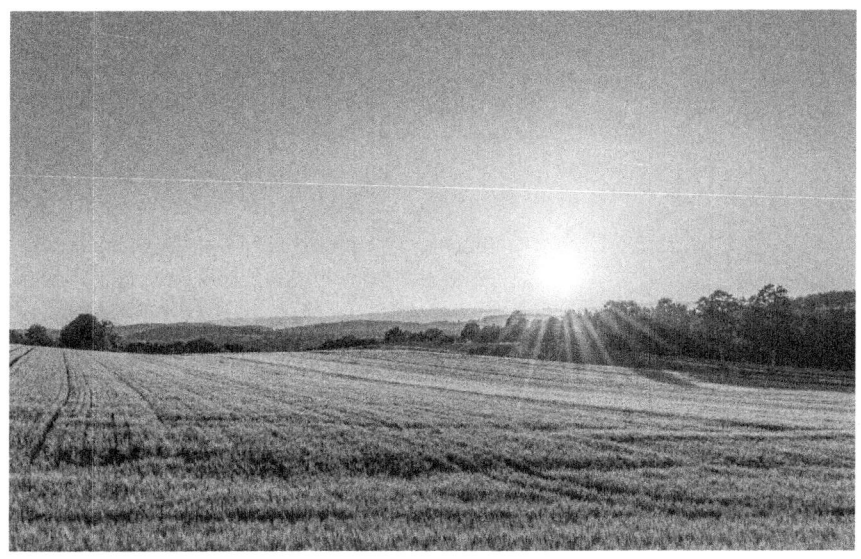

rich in melatonin, such as bananas, pineapples, oranges, oats and walnuts.

Some studies suggest that melatonin enhances cytokine production, thus enhancing immune function. Other studies suggest melatonin is useful in fighting cancer and infectious diseases, including HIV. It regulates over 500 genes and has been shown to be elevated in the blind, which may explain their decreased cancer risk.

Melatonin is synthesised from l-tryptophan, via serotonin production. It is activated in the evening as natural light dims and inhibited by exposure to daylight. Artificial light can disrupt this natural cycle. Blue light suppresses melatonin release, so using glasses that block blue light in the hours before bedtime or adjusting lighting from blue and white to orange and yellow may help reduce melatonin loss and encourage better sleep.

> Circadian disturbances, such as exposure to bright light at night, shift work or travel across time zones, affect melatonin secretion and impact energy metabolism.

Melatonin is also involved in the regulation of energy homeostasis. Melatonin regulates the synthesis and release of leptin (a satiety hormone), as well as its daily rhythmicity, lowering levels at night. Studies in rats have found that melatonin supplementation reduced food intake, body weight and body fat. This effect is thought to be mediated by heightened leptin sensitivity and correlated reduced expression of AgRP and orexin (appetite-stimulating factors). The absence of melatonin is associated with leptin resistance, which lowers our sensitivity to this satiety signal. Circadian disturbances, such as exposure to bright light at night, shift work or travel across time zones, affect melatonin secretion and impact energy metabolism and, consequently, weight.

The release of melatonin also mediates the release of human growth hormone (HGH) during deep sleep, by increasing sensitivity to growth hormone releasing hormone (GHRH). HGH is well known to repair and maintain lean muscle, reduce fat tissue, and improve cognitive and immune function.

Cortisol
Cortisol is a glucocorticoid hormone released by the adrenal glands. It regulates a wide range of processes, including metabolism, blood pressure, immune response and memory function, but it is best known as the stress hormone. Cortisol release is inversely synchronised with melatonin release in order to establish the daily sleep-wake cycle; cortisol wakes us up and melatonin puts us to sleep. Cortisol levels decrease in the evening as melatonin levels increase, inducing tiredness and preparation for sleep. Meanwhile, the onset of daylight increases cortisol levels and decreases melatonin levels, inducing wakefulness and alertness in preparation for a new day.

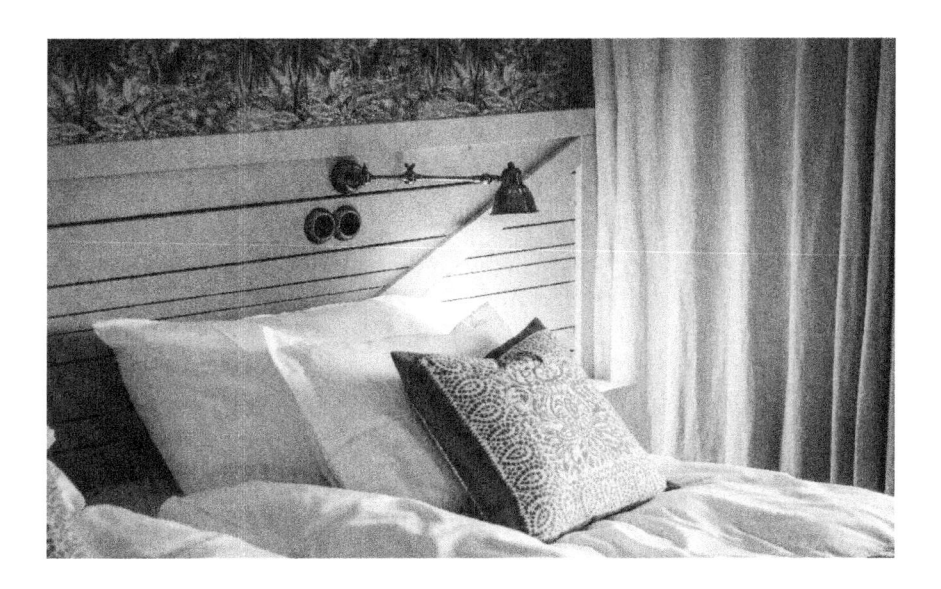

Imbalances in the cortisol/melatonin interplay may cause drowsiness in the morning, insomnia or frequent waking at night. These imbalances may be caused by stress, light exposure from screens or lighting, irregular bedtimes or excessive use of stimulants, such as coffee or sugar.

> Sleep deficiency increases cortisol levels and ghrelin, both of which increase food intake.

Sleep deficiency increases cortisol levels and ghrelin, both of which increase food intake. High cortisol levels in turn will perpetuate and exacerbate disrupted sleep patterns and affect night-time HGH release, which is essential to healthy body composition, immune function and repair in the body. High cortisol levels also cause resistance in hormone receptors to hormones such as insulin, leptin, thyroid, oestrogen, testosterone and to cortisol itself.

Thus, regulation of cortisol levels via good sleep patterns (regular bedtimes and sufficient hours of sleep) and the balancing of stress with relaxing activities, especially in the evening, supports the health-giving attributes of a stable sleep-wake cycle.

Orexin
Orexin is a neuropeptide produced in the hypothalamus that is projected throughout the central nervous system (CNS) to stimulate wakefulness, regulate energy expenditure and modulate visceral function. It is involved in the regulation of HGH, adrenocorticotropic hormone, thyroid, mineralocorticoid and cortisol secretion.

Orexin seems to have an influence over the activation of brown adipose tissue, which uses energy for heat generation (thermogenesis). In studies, orexin-knockout mice displayed reduced brown adipose tissue and therefore reduced thermogenesis as well as increased obesity. A deficiency of orexin is also linked to narcolepsy, a sleep disorder which involves bouts of excessive sleepiness during the day and which is also frequently accompanied by obesity.

In order to activate wakefulness, orexin stimulates the dopamine, noradrenaline, histamine, serotonin and acetylcholine systems. Once activated, orexin promotes wakefulness, increases body temperature, locomotion and energy expenditure.

Orexin is stimulated by ghrelin and low blood glucose levels, while it is inhibited by leptin and high blood glucose levels. Orexin stimulates glucose uptake in fat cells, increasing lipogenesis and inhibiting lipolysis. However, it also increases the secretion of adiponectin, which is involved in fat metabolism.

Sleep deprivation has been linked to increased food intake caused by increased food cravings, which leads to weight gain. Orexin would appear to be a key player in this relationship.

> Sleep deprivation has been linked to increased food intake caused by increased food cravings, which leads to weight gain.

The Purpose of Sleep
The circadian rhythm presupposes a period of sleep, which presupposes a period of fasting every day at least as long as the sleep phase. During the sleep phase, as previously mentioned, the body rests, repairs and regenerates. Cortisol levels fall, melatonin levels increase and the greatest daily surge of human growth hormone (HGH) is released to support this repair and regeneration phase. Every tissue and organ in the body has a circadian rhythm that takes advantage of this sleep phase to switch to an alternate metabolic mode, involving repair in order to be ready for peak performance during the active awake phase.

In order for the circadian rhythm to promote optimum health, all these processes need to be synchronised. However, they can be easily disrupted by late-night studying, working or socialising, travel across time zones, irregular mealtimes, bright lights, loud noises and stress, even irregular bedtimes are enough to throw the circadian rhythm out of sync.

In order to sustain the optimum health of the body, it is essential to respect its circadian rhythm. Activities such as eating, exercising and work should be carried out when the digestive system, cardiovascular system, skeletal muscle system and the brain are all functioning at peak levels during the day. As the evening approaches, these

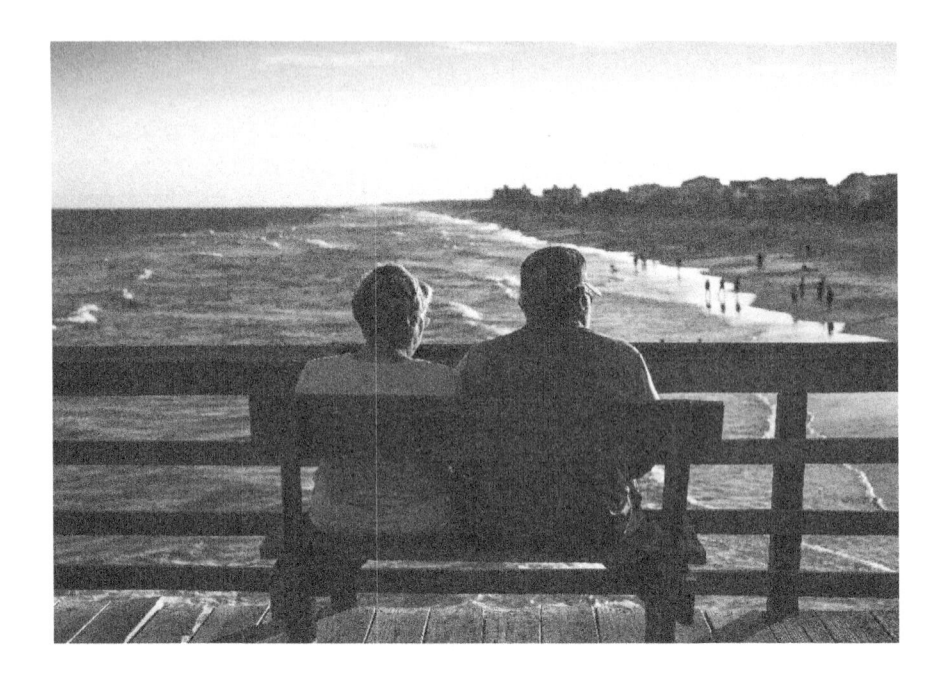

activities should ideally be phased out in order to prepare the body for its night-time phase of rest, repair and regeneration.

The body prepares for each circadian phase by synchronising hormonal release accordingly. Cortisol, insulin and body temperature all decline in the evening in preparation for sleep and rise as morning approaches to prepare the body for waking up and getting active. Similarly, melatonin, HGH, prolactin, antidiuretic hormone and oxytocin surge late in the evening to facilitate sleep and the repair properties of sleep, while they decline as morning approaches.

The shorter the duration of sleep, the higher diurnal levels of ghrelin (a hunger signal) will be and the lower levels of leptin (a satiety signal), which results in higher levels of appetite and food intake. So, there is an inverse relationship between hours of sleep and ghrelin levels and a positive relationship between hours of sleep and leptin levels. Adequate sleep balances ghrelin and leptin levels, rendering excessive food intake and obesity less likely.

As described previously, this cycle is set by exposure to light, but studies have also shown that the peripheral oscillators, in particular in the liver, pancreas and spleen, are more emphatically set by eating patterns. Therefore, in our daily lives, the factors that most categorically reinforce or adjust our circadian rhythm are exposure to light and eating. So, the first exposure to bright light and our first meal restart our clocks on the day cycle. Similarly, in the evening, the dimming of light and the completion of eating herald the night-time mode of our internal clock.

Disruption of the circadian rhythm
The dawn of artificial light meant that it was possible to be active twenty-four hours a day and the progress of technology means that we can be connected to activity and stimulation at all hours of the day and night. If our activity/rest cycle is disrupted, our feeding/fasting cycle usually follows suit. When we stay up longer, sleep less or find our sleep disrupted by modern demands and stresses, feeding no longer becomes confined to set mealtimes.

On average, it is estimated that we are all sleeping 1-2 hours less than

> Sleep deprivation has a negative effect on various hormones related to weight management. Perceptions of satiety decline in individuals who sleep less than 7 hours a night.

50 years ago. Sleep deprivation has a negative effect on various hormones related to weight management. As seen above, sleep deprivation or interrupted sleep cause an imbalance in both leptin and ghrelin levels, which can spiral and, through their effect on eating, further disrupt the circadian rhythm that perpetuates health. Perceptions of satiety decline in individuals who sleep less than 7 hours a night, so their urge to eat is stronger.

A third factor that can disrupt the circadian rhythm along with light and feeding is stress. Chronic stress affects cortisol levels, which we saw previously are a vital regulator together with melatonin of our sleep-wake cycle. If cortisol levels remain high at bedtime, it will be more difficult to fall asleep and sleep may be frequently interrupted. Furthermore, cortisol levels are inversely related to HGH, so high cortisol levels can disrupt the vital repair properties of sleep supported by HGH.

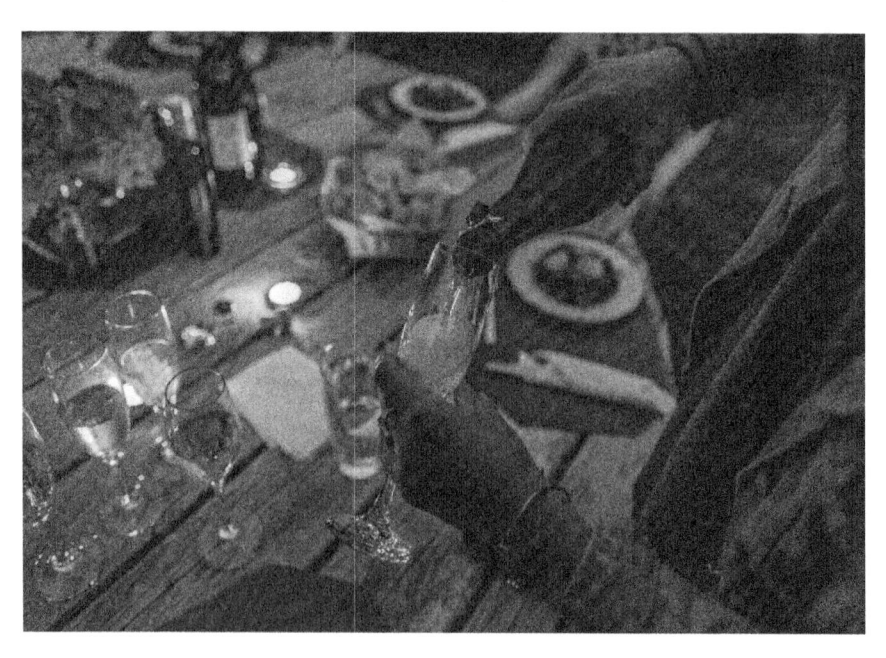

The circadian rhythm can be disrupted by feeding patterns, in particular by eating late at night. Having a late dinner forces all organs that participate in the digestive process to be active at a time when they would otherwise be in repair mode. Insulin sensitivity declines from a peak in the morning to its lowest in the evening. If we eat when our cells are at their most insulin resistant, we are more likely to store the energy consumed as fat rather than utilise it for energy production. Insulin secretion stimulated by food intake also has an inhibitory effect on melatonin and HGH release, which again further inhibits the repair properties of sleep.

Additionally, melatonin receptors are present in pancreatic beta islet cells, so, if melatonin secretion is triggered by the dimming of light, it will inhibit insulin release. Therefore, when we eat late in the evening, blood glucose levels will remain high, inhibiting HGH release, while fuelling systemic inflammation and glycation. Eating also induces thermogenesis, so, if we eat late in the evening, our body temperature is rising at a time when it would be falling in preparation for sleep.

The gastrointestinal tract also functions on a circadian rhythm. In the day phase, it is active with digestion and in the night phase it carries out important repair work. This repair work is vital for maintaining the enteric lining. If we do not respect the circadian rhythm of our gut, by allowing it sufficient respite for repair (at least 12 hours), problems such as leaky gut syndrome, irritable bowel syndrome and acid reflux become more common, fuelling inflammation.

The gut bacteria also operate on a circadian rhythm. The gut environment, including pH levels, varies according to the time of day and what we have eaten, so it promotes the proliferation of different sets of bacteria. Fasting creates a different environment to digestion, so the more we separate the day into distinct fasting and feeding phases, the more diverse our microbiome will be and the healthier our digestive system.

> Both shift work and repeated jet-lag profoundly disrupt the circadian rhythm, reducing melatonin release, causing neuro-hormonal deregulation of appetite and increased risk of obesity, diabetes, insomnia, depression, hypertension, cardiovascular disease and cancer.

10-15% of the protein-encoding genome is regulated by circadian clocks and 40-50% of those genes deal with metabolism. Both shift work and repeated jet-lag profoundly disrupt the circadian rhythm, reducing melatonin release, causing neuro-hormonal deregulation of appetite, including increased ghrelin and decreased leptin levels, insulin resistance, metabolic dysfunction and increased risk of obesity, diabetes, ulcers, reproductive issues, compromised cognitive function, inflammatory conditions, insomnia, depression, hypertension, cardiovascular disease and cancer. Melatonin, in particular, has been shown to inhibit cancer cell growth, stimulate anti-cancer immunity and modulate oncogene expression. Blue and white light suppress melatonin production. So, working on our computers, watching television or using smart phones in the evening can disrupt the onset of our sleep cycle and reduce all the potential benefits of healthy melatonin release.

In studies, night-shift workers, as compared with day-shift workers, had greater body fat mass percentage, greater food intake, impaired sleep, lower insulin sensitivity, increased triglycerides, increased C-reactive protein and blunted post-meal suppression of ghrelin.

Establishing a regular routine, which optimises melatonin release, will ensure high quality sleep with all the regenerative benefits, more mental alertness, vitality and productivity during the day, as well as easier weight management.

Understanding Timing

Understanding the benefits of a daily fasting phase, trying to live in sync with the body's circadian rhythm and practising TRF are clearly beneficial, but how difficult is it to put this lifestyle adjustment into practice? Beyond an adaptation period of a few days, this lifestyle practice becomes easy and natural as it is supported by hormonal changes in the body. Rather than feeling hungrier on TRF, people report feeling less hungry than before when their eating patterns were more irregular. TRF is also far easier than the caloric restriction that has been advocated for decades that rapidly turns into a fight against hunger and a dwindling BMR.

> Beyond an adaptation phase of a few days, this lifestyle practice becomes easy and natural as it is supported by hormonal changes in the body.

Caloric restriction coupled with daily aerobic exercise has been the basis of the majority of dietary advice in the last century. However, as BMR decreases in response to the reduced caloric intake, while hunger signals become overwhelming, this is very difficult advice to follow requiring much willpower. Caloric restriction leads to some weight loss, but once willpower is exhausted, the weight quickly returns. This common cycle of dieting causes BMR to plateaus at successively lower levels and lean muscle mass suffers, so that it becomes increasingly difficult to maintain a stable, healthy weight.

Attention to macronutrient proportions has promised an easier approach; high-fat, low-carbohydrate, high-protein diets have all gone some way to disprove the notion that a calorie is just a calorie. We can all agree that the metabolic effect of a glass of cola is very different to that of a slice of cheese even though they both may contain the same number of calories. Consequently, we now know that our focus should revolve more around which diet delivers the correct amount of nutrients the body requires for optimum health rather than exclusive attention to calories. More understanding regarding the therapeutic impact of certain nutrients and their influence on general health, metabolism and circadian rhythm will be covered in Chapter Three.

Until recently, very few scientists were considering another fundamental parameter of diet, that is, the frequency and timing of meals. However, researchers started to notice that it is not only what you eat that is important; when you eat is of equal importance in the quest for healthy weight management. By just increasing the overnight fast to a duration of at least 12 hours, biomarkers of health are improved. The key to these health benefits is linked to the metabolic shift that occurs during fasting from glucose metabolism to fat metabolism and ketone production, which trigger adaptive cellular stress responses that prevent and repair molecular damage. As soon as glucose and glycogen are depleted, lipolysis is upgraded and free fatty acids are metabolised. Ketones, β-hydroxybutyrate (β-OHB) and acetoacetate, produced from fat metabolism, provide an alternative energy source, inducing mitochondrial biogenesis, reducing oxidative stress and reducing inflammation.

> By just increasing the overnight fast to a duration of 12 hours, biomarkers of health are improved. The key to these health benefits is linked to the metabolic shift that occurs during fasting from glucose metabolism to fat metabolism.

TRF delivers comparable results to caloric restriction in terms of delayed ageing, but exceeds those of caloric restriction in terms of reduced glucose and insulin levels, reduced insulin resistance, reduced inflammation and protection against obesity, hypertension, diabetes, cancer, heart disease, neurodegenerative diseases and fatty liver disease (hepatic steatosis). TRF is also an easier and more reliable weight loss method that favours the maintenance of lean muscle mass and mobilises fat reserves more easily and effortlessly than caloric restriction. TRF is also more efficient at improving the gut microbiota and bile acid profiles, as well as altering liver metabolome to upgrade nutrient absorption and utilisation.

The body tends to thrive on regularity. If the body can prepare for regularly-timed events, such as meals and bedtime, then it is best enabled to work on an alternating rhythmic cycle in which each metabolic phase is optimised. Feeding at different times of day to usual meal times and going to bed at different times each day desynchronises peripheral clocks, makes the body less efficient and can contribute to obesity and metabolic disorders.

The first bite of food in the morning starts the TRF window. It has been proven that benefits accrue just by keeping the feeding window within twelve hours and without any adjustment to the diet. This is an easy first step. Most people tend to cover on average a 15-hour window between breakfast, for example at 7am, and finishing dinner or late-night snacks by 10pm or later. Just reducing this feeding window to twelve hours attenuates the metabolic diseases arising from obesogenic diets and can turn the tide around from escalating weight gain back in the direction of healthy weight management.

The second step after maintaining a 12-hour window is to either improve the diet within the window and/or reduce the window further. Further benefits accrue in proportion to the fasting period and weight loss is enhanced as the feeding window is squeezed down to eight hours. This shorter window may involve a later breakfast, for example at 10am, and all eating completed by 6pm or breakfast at 7am, a mid-morning snack and lunch, then dinner is skipped altogether.

Furthermore, research also shows that the benefits achieved on TRF can be maintained even with a longer feeding window a couple of times a week. This possibility allows us to apply a tighter feeding window during the week and relax it on the weekends, which works well with most lifestyles. It is an easy system to implement as it concedes a greater freedom in application without compromising results.

The fasting period includes time spent asleep. If the feeding window regularly overruns twelve hours, the body spends more time focused on digestion than on repair and renewal, which can result in health issues and weight gain. As the feeding window is reduced below twelve hours, benefits increase ranging from easier weight management to the prevention and enhanced treatment of diseases. Once glucose and glycogen reserves have been exhausted, the body shifts fully into an alternative metabolic phase in which it starts to mobilise fat for energy. A consistent daily shift into fat mobilisation and utilisation rather than the monopoly of glucose as an energy source is highly beneficial for weight management and general health.

> If the feeding window regularly overruns twelve hours, the body spends more time focused on digestion than on repair and renewal, which can result in health issues and weight gain. As the feeding window is reduced below 12 hours, benefits accrue ranging from easier weight management to the prevention and enhanced treatment of diseases.

Disruption of metabolic cycles does not occur solely by eating frequently throughout the day and night, but also by poor sleep habits. Maintaining a normal feeding cycle with a feeding window of less than twelve hours is highly conducive to better sleep patterns and vice-versa; better sleep patterns are also more conducive to better dietary habits. Sleep deprivation reduces energy expenditure and increases food intake, thus has been proven to be a significant driver of obesity and related metabolic conditions, including type 2 diabetes and heart disease, with shift workers being especially vulnerable.

Disrupted sleep may also presuppose reduced melatonin levels. We have seen that melatonin is an essential player in the sleep-wake cycle, but it has also been shown that melatonin delivers potent anti-oxidative protection, improves mitochondrial function, is neuroprotective and increases immune responsiveness. It is thus a key element of the repair and rejuvenation function of sleep. With disrupted sleep and disrupted melatonin release, damage can accumulate and ageing is accelerated with its concomitant chronic degenerative diseases.

We have also seen that melatonin, via receptors in the pancreatic islets, inhibits insulin, so as the body prepares for sleep in the evening, it is less efficient at digesting a meal. However, this is at odds with average meal timing, in which dinner is usually the biggest meal of the day. The body is at its most insulin resistant in the evening and so at its least efficient for metabolising food into energy. It is the time of day, therefore, in which food is most likely to be stored as fat. This effect is compounded by the insulin-inhibiting action of melatonin.

> The body is at its most insulin resistant in the evening and so at its least efficient for metabolising food into energy. It is the time of day, therefore, in which food is most likely to be stored as fat. This effect is compounded by the insulin-inhibiting action of melatonin.

Both eating late in the evening and disrupted sleep diminish the effectiveness of the vital health ally that sleep represents. For the majority of people in developed countries, it is one of the few periods during the day in which eating is absent for long enough in order to trigger a metabolic shift from glucose as a primary fuel source to fat as a primary fuel source. Sleep, coupled with this alternative metabolic system, triggers numerous biological processes of heightened repair, recovery and waste disposal. This night-time mode is a boon for weight management in that, if ushered in correctly, can allow weight loss to occur during sleep. By reinforcing the body's circadian rhythm (through regular sleep and eating patterns) and practising TRF (ensuring that dinner and exposure to bright lights are concluded at least a couple of hours before bedtime), the body will start to support rather than sabotage weight loss. There is no easier or healthier way to lose weight.

TIMING PROTOCOL

Considering what we have learnt in this chapter, the healthiest plan, which is also the most conducive to weight loss and management, is one that respects the body's circadian rhythm as often as possible. Here follow the four steps to put in action right away in order to harness the facilitating power of right timing.

Step One: Start a stopwatch on feeding

Being aware of the timing of your meals is a very easy first step towards effortless weight management. All that is required is an eye on the time.

In order to apply this step today, you will need to ask yourself a simple question:
- At what time did I first eat after waking up?

Once you have this time, add 12 hours to it and you'll have your maximum timeslot for eating all meals. From now on, you are going to keep any eating and drinking (except water) within a maximum time frame of 12 hours. So, if you have your breakfast at 7am, you will finish all eating for the day by 7pm. As often as possible, make sure you complete your last meal a few hours before bedtime.

As with all recommendations in this book, exceptions will arise, but as long as they are kept as exceptions and don't become your normality, your regular habit of respecting the 12-hour window will ensure that you are doing your best to support the body's health, by respecting its cycles and its need for balance, while priming its in-built weight management function.

So, respecting this 12-hour timeslot is beneficial for weight loss as it works in harmony with the body's circadian rhythm. By respecting your body's circadian rhythm, you will be allowing your body to move towards greater health, efficiency and balance. By so doing, your body will support your desire to be in great shape and work with you in your efforts rather than thwarting your best intentions.

Step Two: Narrowing the Window
If you regularly have an eating timeslot of over 12 hours, start today and in the course of a week aim to keep your eating within a timeslot of 12 hours. Once you have acquired the habit of checking your timeslot and making sure you don't go over 12 hours, try reducing this timeslot as often as possible down to 10 hours or 8 hours.

In order to boost weight loss, reducing your feeding window down to 8 hours is an easy step in the right direction. It means that if you are eating your breakfast at 10am, you will finish all eating by 6pm. If you want to keep your breakfast at 7am, for an 8-hour window, you will need to finish eating by 3pm. You can shift the window according to what works best for you and this small commitment alone will already kick-start your weight loss as your body starts to tip the balance between the assimilation of energy from the food you eat to the elimination of stored energy from fat reserves in the body.

Step Three: Dietary Considerations
We will study nutrition in more detail in Chapter Three, but for now consider the following:
- ✓ During your feeding window, eat a balanced and nutritious diet. Start choosing healthy options that nourish your body;
- ✓ Keep the frequency of meals to a maximum of 3 a day (remember that every time you eat, you are triggering the release of insulin, which inhibits fat loss, so it is preferable to eat 2 to 3 satisfying meals rather than 5 to 6 meals or snacks);

- ✓ Eat foods that promote insulin sensitivity, such as those high in fibre, omega-3 fatty acids, vitamin D, carnitine, turmeric, garlic, cinnamon, ginger, green tea, resveratrol, magnesium, chromium, berberine and apple cider vinegar;
- ✓ Eat foods high in melatonin or tryptophan (that can be converted into melatonin), such as eggs, fish, almonds, walnuts, bananas, pineapples, oranges and cherries;
- ✓ Eat your largest meal at lunchtime when the body's digestion and metabolism of food is at its most efficient. Make dinner the lightest meal of the day (or skip altogether if you are narrowing your feeding window to 8 hours) as the body is at its most insulin inefficient in the evening.

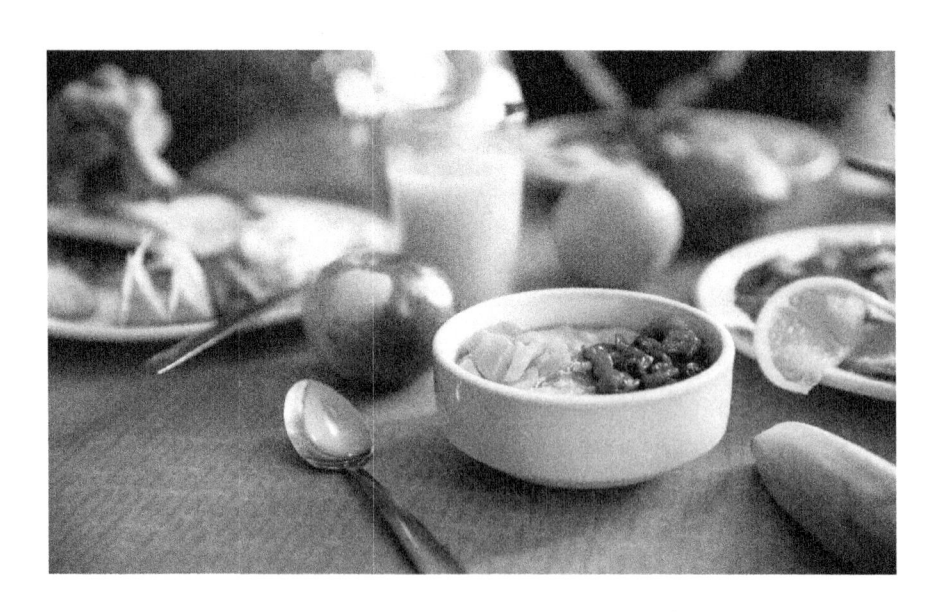

Step Four: A Good Night's Sleep

We have learnt how sleep deprivation is detrimental to weight management; it creates hormonal imbalances that drive over-eating and weight gain. Sleep is also an important daily phase of rest and regeneration to repair the wear and tear on the body simply from being alive, active and breathing. In order to facilitate the best

possible sleep and optimise its repair function, try to integrate as many of the following tips into your routine as possible:
- ✓ Exercise daily (we will learn more about exercise in Chapter Four);
- ✓ Get exposure to bright light in the morning, preferably sunlight;
- ✓ Balance daily stress with stress-relieving activities, such as a relaxing chat with positive friends, meditation, a yoga session, a warm bath, a walk in nature, a feel-good film, a massage or just a break from activity to daydream;
- ✓ Complete all meals by 8pm at the latest (the odd exception is acceptable);
- ✓ Dim lighting in the evenings and reduce screen time to an absolute minimum;
- ✓ Try to keep to a regular bedtime that allows for 8 hours sleep.

The above protocol will rebalance your body and allow for the optimisation of processes conducive to easy weight management. Get into the swing of this timing quadrant of The BODYBLISS Protocol. Its mastery is very easy and its benefits far exceed the commitment required. Having mastered when to eat, we are now ready to understand a little more about why we eat and in particular what subconscious, psychological factors sometimes drive us to eat beyond our needs.

Chapter Two – MINDSET

Appetite is regulated by physiological cues of hunger, but we don't only eat when we are hungry. Sometimes appetite is stimulated by exposure to appetising foods, sometimes we eat because it is dinnertime and sometimes we eat because we are triggered by psychological cues.

> The opposing neurological and endocrinological signals of hunger and satiety tend to perpetuate weight management, as long as they are functioning optimally and other factors do not knock these signals off balance.

The opposing neurological and endocrinological signals of hunger and satiety tend to perpetuate weight management, as long as they are functioning optimally and other factors (that we will explore in the rest of this book and some that we have seen already, such as poor timing) do not knock these signals off balance.

Hunger is defined as our desire to eat and satiety is the satisfaction of this desire, it is the sensation of fullness or sufficiency that increases our desire to stop rather than continue eating. Ordinarily and optimally speaking, when energy reserves are running low in the body, hunger signals are triggered that urge us to eat, but as soon as we have eaten sufficiently, satiety signals take over to reduce our desire to continue eating. Psychological factors can tip this self-regulating system off balance and push us to ignore hunger signals or eat beyond our hunger, driving us towards excessive weight loss or gain respectively.

Again, if you would like to cut straight to the chase and start implementing the mindset principles for optimum weight management, go straight to the end of this chapter to the section entitled "**MINDSET PROTOCOL**". Otherwise, to learn the science relevant to how your mind affects weight management, read on.

The Physiology and Psychology of Appetite

The principal assumption in this topic is that a factor of weight gain is the excessive intake of food. For the moment, we will leave aside diet composition or a subject's greater or lesser tendency to gain weight and the factors upon which that depends, and focus solely on the nature of our urge to eat. Again, unlike so many other diet manuals, this book maintains that **when** and now **why** you eat are as important as **what** you eat.

> Unlike so many other diet manuals, this book maintains that **when** and **why** you eat are as important as **what** you eat.

The assumption that excessive food intake results in excess body weight necessitates the analysis of both the desire to eat and the desire to stop eating, that is, hunger and satiety. We will explore the factors involved in the brain's regulation of appetite and its effects upon the regulation of food intake and whether any tools exist to limit the excessive appetite that can contribute to weight gain.

Weight management is facilitated by food intake regulation and it is rendered difficult by excessive hunger or an excessive desire to eat, where the two terms are not always synonymous, but rather the former is considered a purely physiological stimulus and the latter has an added psychological inducement. We will explore both aspects in this chapter on mindset.

The body tends to maintain energy balance and subsequently weight balance by modulating neurological and endocrinological hunger signals to regulate energy input according to the distribution of energy between energy production, heat production and energy reserves of glycogen and fat.

The psychological factors that affect our eating habits are controlled by different neuronal circuits to the physiological cues of hunger and satiety. They are characterised by patterns of motivation and reward and play out mainly in the limbic system and cerebral cortex, whereas physiological factors are mainly headquartered in the hypothalamus.

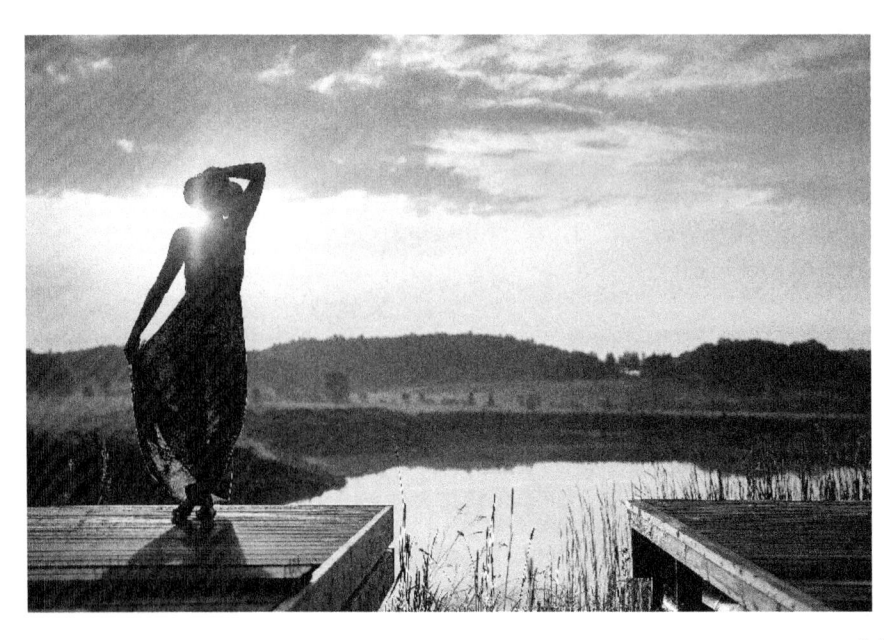

In order to attain and sustain our ideal weight, it is absolutely essential to address these, often subconscious, factors that frequently sabotage our intentions. It may be that your emotional state does not affect your eating behaviour, but, if so, you are one of the few. We will look at the varying degrees of how emotions can affect behaviour and ways to offset the negative impact of emotional eating.

We will also look at how, in your quest for optimum health and ideal weight, your mind can be your best ally instead of your own worst enemy. The psychological component of weight is really important, it will inform your food choices and affect your decision-making, so any weight management programme that does not take this component into account is flawed from the outset and doomed to failure in the long run.

But first, let's cover all the physiological elements of why we eat.

The Need to Feed
The sensation of hunger is a necessary physiological impulse as it ensures that the body prioritises eating enough to provide a sufficient energy intake to sustain metabolic needs. The existence of the sensation of hunger keeps us alive; it is a force of survival, it renders the importance of fuelling our bodies sufficiently overriding that we are unlikely not to eat if we feel the urge to do so and food is available, unless we override our hunger with an equally strong force of self-restriction.

Energy balance is a tightly regulated system in the body. Food intake can vary from day to day and from meal to meal, but, over time, the body seeks to match energy intake with expenditure in order to maintain body weight at a set point. The gauges of hunger and satiety act to provide the necessary action, that is, to eat and to stop eating respectively, that results in weight maintenance.

From an evolutionary perspective as a species, appetite is as essential to our survival as reproduction. We are hard-wired to seize opportunities to replenish and add to energy stores in the body in order to safeguard against periods during which the availability of food may be restricted. The sight, smell and taste of food incite our appetite, rendering us more likely to take advantage of every occasion to add to our energy stores. Eating is also reinforced by hedonic reward pathways in the brain, which can drive the desire to eat beyond purely biological needs.

Where food is plentiful, as is the case in the developed world, the constant availability of food and our evolutionary tendency to take advantage of every opportunity to eat in order to store up fat for times of scarcity, create an equation that often results in weight gain and obesity. We will investigate how effective appetite is in controlling energy intake in an environment where the opportunity to eat is omnipresent and our constant sensorial bombardment with appetising food becomes an irresistible trigger.

> The constant availability of food and our evolutionary tendency to take advantage of every opportunity to eat in order to store up fat for times of scarcity, create an equation that often results in weight gain and obesity.

Furthermore, eating has become such an ingrained socio-cultural habit that, whether driven by appetite or not, most people mark their days with regular meals, the most common pattern being breakfast, lunch and dinner, often with a number of snacks in between.

Even when we regulate our eating by predetermined mealtimes rather than the call of appetite, we will study what affects how much we eat at each sitting. In effective weight management, whether a subject has two big meals a day or six, the stimulus provided by satiety is a safety gauge that can contribute significantly to keeping weight within healthy parameters.

Most diets aimed at weight loss provide calorie-restricted meal plans that rely heavily on the subject's willpower to both contain the urge to eat and defy the absence of satiety. The strength of physiological urges can override willpower and systematically sabotage the long-term success of such diets.

> Most diets aimed at weight loss provide calorie-restricted meal plans that rely heavily on the subject's willpower to both contain the urge to eat and defy the absence of satiety. The strength of physiological urges can override willpower and systematically sabotage the long-term success of such diets.

First, then, we will seek to understand the factors involved in appetite control, that is, the biological processes that determine the oscillating balance between hunger and satiety, and then we will study the most effective tools to support appetite control for healthy weight management.

The Inverse Relationship between Hunger and Satiety
Hunger cancels out signals of satiety in the body and vice-versa. This oscillation is regulated by the interplay between signals from the gastrointestinal tract, fat cells and the brain.

Hunger, the desire to eat, is physiologically triggered by the following orexigenic (appetite-stimulating) factors:
- Neuropeptide Y (NPY)
- Agouti-related peptide (AgRP)
- Orexins (A, B)
- Melanin-concentrating hormone (MCH)
- Sensory stimuli
- Ghrelin

- Low levels of glucose, amino acids and fatty acids
- Low levels of insulin and leptin
- High levels of glucagon

Satiety, the absence of hunger or desire to eat, is triggered by the following anorexigenic (appetite-reducing) factors:
- Pro-opiomelanocortin (POMC) and (α,β,γ)-Melanocyte-stimulating hormones (MSH)
- Cocaine- and amphetamine-regulated transcript (CART)
- Corticotropin-releasing hormone (CRH)
- Cholecystokinin (CCK)
- Pancreatic Peptide (PP)
- Peptide YY (PYY)
- Glucagon-like peptide – 1 (GLP-1)
- Oxyntomodulin (OXM)
- High levels of glucose, amino acids and fatty acids
- High levels of insulin and leptin
- Low levels of glucagon

Appetite Control Centre

Appetite is controlled in the hypothalamus, the regulator of the autonomic nervous system (ANS), which also regulates thirst, sleep, circadian rhythm, blood pressure, heart rate, digestion, respiratory rate, bonding, body temperature, memory and learning. The autonomic nervous system functions without any conscious effort or control from us and comprises two antagonistic sets of nerves: the sympathetic nervous system (the fight-or-flight system) and the parasympathetic nervous system (the feed-and-breed or rest-and-digest system).

The hypothalamus responds to signals it receives, such as:
- Daylight for circadian rhythm regulation;
- Stress;
- Bacterial and viral infections by resetting the body's thermostat upward to increase body temperature;
- Sensorial stimuli;

- Hormones, such as leptin, ghrelin and insulin;
- Steroids;
- Vagus nerve stimuli, such as cardiovascular signals and gastric distension;

Appetite is modulated by a cluster of neurons in the hypothalamus called the arcuate nucleus (ARC). The ARC contains two distinct neuron populations that together regulate appetite. The ARC's prime purpose is homeostasis through its influence on feeding, metabolism, fertility and cardiovascular regulation.

The ARC is accessible to circulating appetite modulators due to its position at the base of the hypothalamus where the blood-brain barrier (BBB) is semi-permeable. Long-term signals that communicate fluctuations in health and body composition and short-term signals that communicate fluctuations in energy intake and expenditure from the periphery lead to the expression of either the pro-opiomelanocortin (POMC) and cocaine- and amphetamine-regulated transcript (CART) anorexigenic expressing neurons or the neuropeptide Y (NPY) and agouti-related peptide (AgRP) orexigenic co-expressing neurons, thus respectively inhibiting food intake and increasing energy expenditure or promoting food intake and reducing energy expenditure, that is, stimulating feelings of satiety or hunger.

Short-term Signals of Hunger and Satiety
Certain short-term signals of hunger and satiety reach the brain from the gastrointestinal tract via vagal nerve fibres. Gastric mechanoreceptors allow the brain to register when the stomach is empty, prompting an activation of hunger, or it registers a signal of distension in the gastrointestinal tract and consequently inhibits appetite. Chemoreceptors register changes in nutrient composition and pH level. The signals terminate in the nucleus of the solitary tract (NTS), which then projects to the hypothalamus.

The hypothalamus thus senses nutrient and energy levels absorbed from the food we eat and adjusts appetite accordingly. Blood levels of glucose, amino acids and fatty acids are registered in the brain; high levels stimulate satiety, low levels stimulate hunger. Desensitisation of these signals is seen in obese subjects and is a cause of habitual overeating, increased meal size and duration.

In Chapter Three, we will study diet composition and macro- and micronutrient modulation and its effects on appetite control and more broadly on weight management.

Gastrointestinal Hormonal Signals
The gastrointestinal tract contains various endocrine cells, which synthesise and secrete appetite-modulating hormones in response to food intake. These hormones provide short-term signals that regulate the urge to eat and the urge to stop eating.

These short-term hormones include ghrelin, the only known orexigenic (appetite-stimulating) gut hormone, and the anorexigenic (satiety-stimulating) cholecystokinin (CCK), pancreatic polypeptide (PP), peptide YY (PYY), glucagon-like peptide (GLP)-1 and oxyntomodulin (OXM). More long-term signals are provided by insulin and leptin.

> Ghrelin levels are negatively correlated with weight, which suggests that ghrelin, like leptin, acts as an adiposity signal. So, the greater our fat reserves, the lower our ghrelin levels, thus reducing our appetite, reducing our food intake and reducing our weight.

Ghrelin
Ghrelin is an orexigenic (appetite-stimulating) peptide hormone synthesised and released by ghrelinergic cells mainly in the stomach when it is empty. When the stomach is full, secretion stops. Ghrelin cells are also found in the jejunum, duodenum, lungs, pancreatic islets, gonads, adrenal cortex, placenta, kidneys and also in the brain.

The typically expected post-prandial fall in circulating ghrelin levels is attenuated, or even absent in the obese, suggestive of a role of ghrelin in the pathophysiology of obesity. However, generally, ghrelin levels are inversely correlated with weight, which suggests that ghrelin, like leptin, acts as an adiposity signal. So, the greater our fat reserves, the lower our ghrelin levels, thus reducing our appetite, reducing our food intake and reducing our weight.

Pharmacological blockage of ghrelin in rodents has been shown to result in decreases in food intake, foraging for food, hoarding of food and body weight. Ghrelin deficient or ghrelin receptor-deficient rodents are resistant to diet-induced obesity.

Ghrelin levels fall more in response to protein consumption than to carbohydrate and lipid consumption. High-protein meals also slow down gastric emptying and prolong the perception of fullness.

Ghrelin inhibits the secretion of gonadotropin-releasing hormone (GnRH), luteinizing hormone (LH), follicle-stimulating hormone (FSH), progesterone and testosterone and so high levels can have a detrimental effect on male and female fertility. This is a mechanism by which calorie-restricted diets can compromise fertility.

Ghrelin levels are inversely related to hours of sleep, with lack of sleep increasing ghrelin levels and reducing leptin levels, which increases hunger signals. This mechanism may be a contributing factor to the link between sleep deprivation and obesity. Ghrelin levels are also higher in people with a vitamin D deficiency.

> Ghrelin levels are inversely related to hours of sleep, with lack of sleep increasing ghrelin levels and reducing leptin levels, which increases hunger signals.

Ghrelin has been attributed anti-depressant and anti-anxiety properties and is up-regulated by stress. Ghrelin has also been shown in animal tests to improve learning and memory, especially Pavlovian fear-conditioned learning. We are more alert to eating opportunities when ghrelin levels are high.

Cholecystokinin

Cholecystokinin (CCK) is a peptide hormone released by hypothalamic neurons as well as enteroendocrine cells in the duodenum and jejunum. CCK release is stimulated most by the presence of fatty acids and certain amino acids in the chime entering the duodenum. It stimulates the release of digestive enzymes and bile from the pancreas and gallbladder respectively, as well as inhibiting gastric emptying and decreasing gastric acid secretion. It is inhibited by somatostatin.

CCK inhibits appetite by activating POMC/CART neurons and dampening NPY/AgRP neurons, thus opposing the effects of ghrelin.

Pancreatic Polypeptide

Pancreatic polypeptide (PP) is secreted by PP cells in the pancreatic islets of Langerhans and to a lesser degree in the colon and rectum. Its main function is to regulate pancreatic endocrine and exocrine secretions, but it also has an effect on motility in the gastrointestinal tract.

> PP levels increase most after a high-protein meal.

Levels of PP increase after eating to induce satiety and reduce food intake, while PP levels fall during fasting to facilitate appetite. PP levels increase most after a high-protein meal, with CCK and gastrin proving potent stimuli. Ghrelin and somatostatin are inhibitors of PP.

PP release is lower in obese subjects. One study showed that when individuals were administered PP, their food intake at a free-choice buffet meal was reduced by 21.8% and this reduction was maintained until the following day.

Peptide YY (PYY)

Peptide YY (PYY) is released after a meal, principally by the L-cells in the mucosa of the gastrointestinal tract. It crosses the BBB and simultaneously inhibits NPY release and stimulates POMC release in the ARC, inducing satiety. It also inhibits gastric motility and gastric emptying, which facilitates better digestion and nutrient absorption, while prolonging the sensation of fullness. PYY is inhibited by stress. Circulating PYY levels have been found to be lower in obese subjects.

Glucagon-like Peptide – 1

Glucagon-like peptide-1 (GLP-1) is a peptide hormone secreted after eating by intestinal enteroendocrine L-cells and certain neurons within the nucleus of the solitary tract in the brainstem. Its effects are anorexigenic (reduce appetite) and reduce food intake, gastric secretion and motility. Slower digestion slows down glucose absorption, reduces insulin spikes and lowers the risk of hypoglycemia.

GLP-1 promotes the secretion of insulin in a glucose-dependent manner, while suppressing glucagon secretion and this action is preserved in type 2 diabetics. In both type 1 and type 2 diabetes, a reduction in functional β-cells is seen; GLP-1 can help this problem as it promotes insulin gene transcription, mRNA stability and biosynthesis, thus increasing β-cell numbers by stimulating proliferation and neogenesis while inhibiting apoptosis. GLP-1 enhances the glucose sensitivity of pancreatic cells, thus enhancing the insulin and glucagon response to glucose levels.

In the brain, GLP-1 decreases appetite, decreases the quantity and frequency of food intake, decreases the hedonic/reward value of food, increases taste aversions and nausea, as well as exerting neurotrophic and neuroprotective effects, including neurogenesis, reduced necrotic and apoptotic signalling and protection against stroke and Alzheimer's disease. GLP-1 has also been studied for its protective properties in other tissues, including the bones, the heart, muscles, liver, kidneys and lungs.

Oxyntomodulin (OXM)
Oxyntomodulin (OXM) is a peptide hormone co-secreted with GLP-1 by intestinal L-cells following feeding. It binds to the GLP-1 receptor and the glucagon receptor and it inhibits appetite, reducing food intake and increasing energy expenditure.

Insulin
As we learnt in the last chapter, insulin is a peptide hormone produced by β-cells in the islets of Langerhans of the pancreas. Beta cells are glucose-sensitive, so when blood glucose levels rise, they secrete insulin into the blood. Insulin lowers blood glucose levels, by shuttling the glucose into cells of insulin-sensitive tissues, such as skeletal muscle cells, liver cells and fat cells.

When blood sugar levels fall, adjacent alpha cells secrete glucagon into the blood to increase blood sugar levels. These opposing processes work together to maintain glucose homeostasis, that is, blood glucose balance, essential to the function of key organs, including the brain, liver and kidneys.

The islets of Langerhans also contain delta cells, which secrete somatostatin that inhibits alpha and beta cells. They also contain gamma cells, which secrete PP.

> Low levels of insulin and glucose promote catabolism (breakdown), especially of fat stores.

Insulin regulates the metabolism of macronutrients by promoting their absorption from the blood into a) fat cells, where they are converted into fat via lipogenesis, b) into liver cells, where they are converted into glycogen via glycogenesis and fat via lipogenesis, and c) into tissue cells, where they are converted into energy. Insulin is, therefore, an anabolic hormone. Low levels of insulin and glucose promote catabolism, especially of fat stores and glycogen stores in the liver, and stimulate the release of glucagon, which increases glucose levels through glycogenolysis or gluconeogenesis in the liver.

Insulin inhibits NPY/AgRP co-expressing orexigenic neurons in the ARC, thus reducing appetite and food intake. Insulin stimulates the synthesis and secretion of leptin from white adipose tissue via the adipo-insular axis feedback loop. As with leptin, insulin levels rise as body fat levels rise, in order to reduce appetite, but can lead to insulin resistance, which further increases excess body fat and both leptin and insulin resistance.

> As with leptin, insulin levels rise as body fat levels rise, and can lead to insulin resistance, which further increases excess body fat and both leptin and insulin resistance.

Insulin has been shown to inhibit autophagy, improve learning and memory, as well as stimulating gonadotropin-releasing hormone from the hypothalamus, thus enhancing fertility. However, together with glucagon, insulin's main role is to keep blood glucose levels stable and to deliver fuel to cells.

Most cells can use other fuels (mainly fatty acids) in the absence of glucose. However, cells that do not contain mitochondria, such as red blood cells, cannot use other fuel sources. Once glucose is depleted, glucagon activates the release of glycogen to provide a short-term reserve of glucose. When glycogen reserves have been depleted, the cells that cannot switch to fatty acids or ketone bodies for fuel, require that glucose be produced from glycerol (the triglyceride backbone of fat), glucogenic amino acids, such as alanine and glutamine, or from pyruvate in a process called gluconeogenesis.

Most cells, with the notable exception of liver cells, require insulin to be able to receive blood glucose. These cells starve when there is an absence of insulin, as occurs for example in type 1 diabetes, or there is a decrease in the sensitivity of cells to insulin, such as occurs with insulin resistance and is a characteristic for example of type 2 diabetes. Both conditions produce hyperglycaemia (elevated blood glucose levels).

Insulin Resistance
The pathology of insulin resistance, in which cells become increasingly insensitive to insulin, is attributed to overstimulation. Excess insulin activation from overeating renders cells progressively less sensitive and less able to transport nutrients from the blood into the cells. This creates hyperglycaemia, which activates the release of more insulin, which further exacerbates the insulin resistance of cells. If this compensatory insulin secretion fails to lower blood glucose levels, eventually type 2 diabetes develops.

As we saw previously, fat cells tend to retain their insulin sensitivity beyond the insulin resistance of skeletal muscle cells, so insulin resistance pours excess blood glucose into fat cells for storage, which accelerates weight gain. The development of insulin resistance in fat cells results in reduced uptake of glucose and lipids and, thus, elevated levels in blood plasma. High levels of lipids in the blood increase their accumulation within muscle tissue. This exacerbates insulin resistance through the activation of protein kinase C, which reduces the ability of the insulin receptor substrates to associate and activate PI 3-kinase, resulting in decreased activation of glucose transport activity.

> Diet composition, in particular, a preference for energy-dense, highly palatable foods and sugary beverages, is the main risk factor for insulin resistance; other factors include a sedentary lifestyle and constant snacking, which stimulates a continual insulinic response.

The continual activation of insulin through high blood

glucose levels, continual over-eating and low energy expenditure, further fuels the vicious cycle that escalates into obesity. Diet composition, in particular, a preference for energy-dense, highly palatable foods and sugary beverages, is a main risk factor for insulin resistance; other factors include a sedentary lifestyle and constant snacking, which stimulates a continual insulinic response.

Dietary restriction combined with regular physical exercise is the most effective therapy to reverse this situation by clearing insulin and excess fuel reserves. Then glucagon and adiponectin levels need to increase such that lipolysis is activated and the excess fat storage and chronic insulin resistance can be reversed.

Some natural substances such as curcumin, resveratrol, vitamin D, capsaicin, gingerol and catechins have been found to increase adiponectin expression. These substances, in particular curcumin, also have potent anti-inflammatory properties that have been shown to sensitise insulin signalling.

Leptin
Leptin is a hormone secreted principally by fat cells in response to food intake and fat levels in the body. It informs the brain regarding the quantity of fat stores in peripheral tissues and simultaneously inhibits NPY/AgRP neurons and stimulates POMC/CART neurons in the hypothalamic ARC to reduce appetite and food intake and increase energy expenditure. Leptin is the main peripheral hormonal stimulus to arcuate POMC neurons. Its action is opposed by the hormone ghrelin. Mutations in the leptin gene, leptin deficiencies and leptin receptor abnormalities have been linked to obesity and hyperphagia (extreme sensation of hunger accompanied by overeating).

Circulating levels of leptin are proportional to total body fat mass and, therefore, are a key component in the regulation of long-term hunger and energy homeostasis by serving as the brain's sensor of the body's total energy reserves. Thus, a rise in fat reserves increases

> A rise in fat reserves increases leptin production, which reduces appetite and consquently food intake.

leptin production, reducing appetite to reduce food intake, and vice versa regarding a fall in fat reserves.

However, most obese subjects have high leptin levels, and yet these do not effectively reduce food intake or reverse weight gain. This is because leptin levels vary exponentially, not linearly, with fat mass and, therefore, increases in food intake and fat stores lead to higher than proportional leptin level increases, which over-stimulate leptin receptors and thus activate negative feedback loops that serve to block leptin signalling. The resulting resistance to leptin prevents increases in leptin from reducing food intake and increases susceptibility to obesity, which in turn increases leptin levels further and exacerbates the existing leptin resistance leading to a vicious cycle of weight gain.

Therefore, leptin is more effective at signalling for weight loss than signalling for weight gain. This may be an evolutionary strength in order to strongly signal potential starvation and the need to conserve fat stores for survival. A day of fasting already significantly decreases leptin levels, even before there has been any change in fat reserves.

A reduction in food intake and fat reserves or an increase in physical exercise causes a disproportionately large drop in leptin levels. This triggers the brain (stimulating NPY/AgRP and inhibiting POMC/CART) to increase appetite, reduce energy expenditure and seek reward-related behaviour (eating and nesting). This is a scenario familiar to dieters, who start with high motivation to reduce food intake and increase exercise, but then find it increasingly difficult to control appetite and engage in physical exercise as they fight against these physiological cues.

These physiological cues triggered by leptin are regulated through leptin receptors (Ob-R) distributed throughout the body and in particular in the brain. The most concentrated region of uptake is the hypothalamic ARC. Access to this region may be impaired by hypertriglyceridemia, a condition induced by insulin resistance and a junk food diet high in carbohydrates.

> Dieters start with high motivation to reduce food intake and increase exercise and then find it increasingly difficult to control appetite and engage in physical exercise as they fight against physiological cues.

Leptin acts directly on leptin receptors in the hypothalamus, in the hippocampus, and in the solitary nucleus (SN) of the brainstem. Leptin signalling regulates bone metabolism, the inflammatory response, white blood cell count and the immune response. Leptin also mediates the effects of insulin, glucagon, insulin-like growth factor, growth hormone, glucocorticoids, cytokines and metabolites. It has an effect on memory, learning and neuroplasticity (low levels of leptin have been linked to depression and Alzheimer's disease), cardiovascular health, blood pressure and it promotes fertility by stimulating the release of gonadotropin-releasing hormone.

The Psychology of Eating

At the end of this chapter, you will find the necessary steps to best balance the above physiological cues to facilitate weight management. We will now turn our attention to the psychological aspects of appetite.

Emotional Eating

Weight gain is broadly caused by consistently eating in excess of the body's energetic requirements. Simply put, we gain weight when we eat more in a certain time frame than the body needs. The body copes with the excess by storing it as fat. Usually a series of signals trigger the sensation of satiety or fullness and lead us to stop eating. Certain foods may delay satiety, but the main reason we overeat is that there are behavioural impulses that override our satiety. The root of these impulses is emotional.

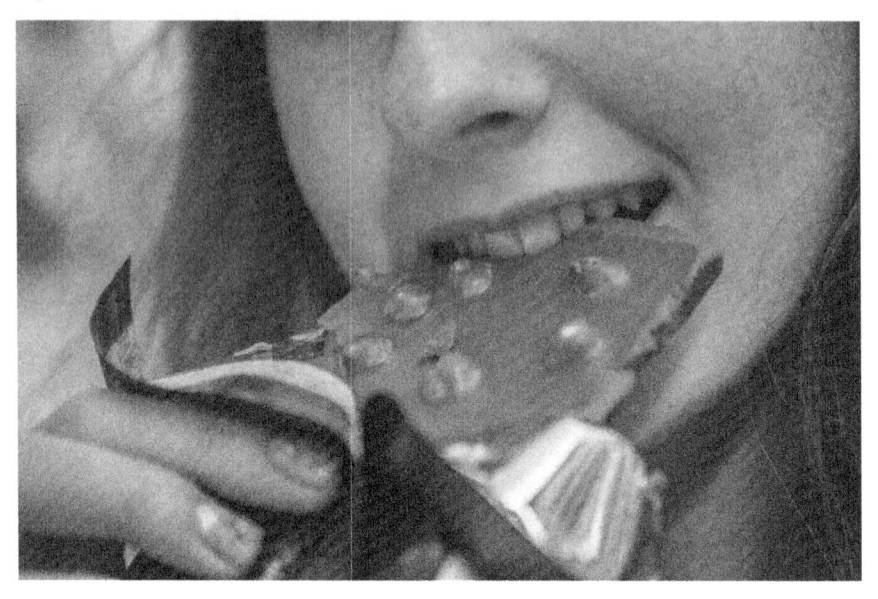

Emotional eating refers to the use of food to manage or numb emotions. Emotional eating encompasses any eating that is triggered by one or more of the following emotional states:

- Stress, fear and anxiety;
- Depression;
- Avoidance, whether of responsibilities, social interaction or intimacy;
- Helplessness: anger, frustration, self-sabotage or low self-esteem;
- Emptiness: sadness, loneliness or boredom;
- Emotional exhaustion, tiredness and lack of sleep.

The consequences of emotional eating depend upon the frequency with which bouts occur and can range from slight weight gain to obesity. However, first let us consider why, when we are usually cognisant of the results of emotional eating, do we still feel compelled to eat beyond all signals of physiological satiety?

The Amygdala – Emotional Control Centre

If eating has an emotional input, we can trace its source to the amygdala, which, once activated, projects onto the hypothalamus, the appetite-regulating centre of the brain, and to the brainstem, also associated with appetite and food intake.

The amygdala is composed of two groups of nuclei located in the temporal lobes of the brain. It forms a part of the limbic system and carries out a primary role in decision-making, emotional reactions and the processing of memory. Studies have shown that the right amygdala is specifically associated with negative emotions, such as fear and sadness, and the left amygdala is associated with both negative and positive emotions, such as happiness. It is hypothesised, therefore, that the left amygdala is involved in the brain's reward system pathways.

The amygdala forms and stores memories associated with emotional events. The greater the emotional content of the information, the greater the amygdala activity and subsequent retention of that information. These emotional memories form the basis of how we react to present stimuli, so that we might pair apparently neutral stimuli with fear due to conditioning by specific emotional memories. Sensory neurons project to the central nucleus of the amygdala, from where many fear responses originate, such as fight-or-flight changes in blood pressure, heart rate and the release of stress hormones.

> Emotional memories form the basis of how we react to present stimuli, so that we might pair apparently neutral stimuli with fear due to conditioning by specific emotional memories.

The two sides of the amygdala work together to process stimuli and produce an emotional response based upon conscious or unconscious associations made with relevant memories. This emotional response conditions the individual to avoid or seek the stimulus in question.

The amygdala, therefore, plays a pivotal role in mental states and is implicated in many psychological disorders. Abnormal levels of activity, underdevelopment or damage to the amygdala have been seen to correlate with anxiety disorders, obsessive compulsive disorders, post traumatic stress disorder (PTSD), borderline personality disorder, bipolar disorder, reduced maternal bonding, physical abuse and neglect.

Stress

The stress response originates in the amygdala. Stress is the body's reaction to an emotional or physical challenge. It is a survival instinct that allows us to respond effectively to danger by facing the challenge or escaping from it. Two opposing branches of the autonomic nervous system (ANS) manage the response to stress and the return to normality. The sympathetic nervous system (SNS) is triggered into fight-or-flight mode by acute stress, while the parasympathetic nervous system (PSNS) is responsible for restoring balance after the trigger has passed, returning the body to rest-and-digest or feed-and-breed mode. As we learnt earlier, the ANS is regulated by the hypothalamus, which is also the appetite control centre of the body.

> Stress is the body's reaction to an emotional or physical challenge. It is a survival instinct that allows us to respond effectively to danger by facing the challenge or escaping from it.

When the amygdala processes incoming information as dangerous, it initiates the stress response. It projects instantaneous distress signals to the hypothalamus. The hypothalamus immediately activates the SNS via the sympathomedullary pathway (SAM), sending signals through the autonomic nerves to the adrenal glands, which immediately start pumping adrenaline and noradrenaline into the bloodstream, which causes the following physiological changes:

- Increased heart rate and force contraction;
- Increased blood pressure and pulse rate;
- Vasoconstriction in many parts of the body and dilation of blood vessels in muscles;
- Bronchodilation;
- Glycogenolysis, gluconeogenesis and lipolysis (for increased energy requirements);
- Sweating and shaking;
- Tunnel vision and dilation of pupils (mydriasis);
- Decreased motility of the digestive system; and
- Relaxation of the bladder wall.

During the stress response, resources for highly demanding metabolic processes, such as digestion and immune function, are diverted to rapid breathing, blood flow, mental alertness and muscle use.

This response is so fast that it allows immediate action in response to the danger, for example, in defending oneself against attack or from an oncoming object, without conscious thought. After this initial surge of adrenaline release, if the perception of danger is still present, the hypothalamus activates a secondary stress response mediated by the hypothalamus-pituitary-adrenal (HPA) axis. This HPA axis also regulates the central nervous system, the cardiovascular system, digestion, metabolism, the immune system, mood and emotions, the reproductive system and energy balance.

If the perception of danger continues, neurons in the paraventricular nucleus (PVN) of the hypothalamus release vasopressin (a vasoconstrictor and anti-diuretic hormone) and corticotropin-releasing hormone (CRH), which stimulates the release of adrenocorticotropic hormone (ACTH) from the pituitary gland, which in turn stimulates the release of glucocorticoid hormones, mainly cortisol, from the adrenal cortex. Cortisol increases catecholamine (adrenaline and noradrenaline) production in the adrenal medulla, which creates a positive feedback loop to the pituitary, increasing the cleavage of POMC into ACTH and β-endorphins. This system is thus able to maintain a state of high alert in the body beyond the initial adrenal activation through the SAM.

Systems involved in the regulation of the stress response and of energy balance are highly integrated. Sustained release of glucocorticoids intensifies the glucose, fat and amino acid mobilisation and concentration in the blood, increasing anorexigenic signals, which strongly inhibit appetite, but this state cannot be fuelled indefinitely. It is followed by exhaustion and the need for recovery.

When the perception of danger passes or the source of stress is normalised or there is adaptation to the challenge, the PSNS takes over to dampen the stress response. At this point, the high levels of glucose, fatty acids and amino acids in the blood are used anabolically to restore balance and regenerate cells. Descending glutaminergic and GABAergic pathways from the amygdala and noradrenergic projections suppress vasopressin and CRH secretion in the hypothalamus and ACTH production in the pituitary gland.

> Both acute and chronic stress can affect weight management by disrupting the catecholamine system, the hypothalamic-pituitary-adrenocortical axis and the serotonin system.

Stress can be sudden and short-lived or low-grade and continuous. Both acute and chronic stress can affect weight management by disrupting the catecholamine system, the hypothalamic-pituitary-adrenocortical axis and the serotonin system. Acute stress can have long-term effects, but it is usually the on-going, daily stress, for example of living in a dangerous neighbourhood, in an abusive marriage or in a stressful job, that has more profound, sustained effects on our physiology. Such chronic stress and a lack of coping strategies can lead to more long-term issues, such as insomnia, anxiety and depression, as well as increasing our vulnerability to illness due to a weakened immune system.

An individual's ability to cope with stress and swiftly return to a state of equilibrium or homeostasis is an important factor in the effect of stress on the body, in terms of general health and weight management.

Let's now analyse in more detail how stress affects eating habits. Firstly, the fight-or-flight response inhibits appetite, which is part of the rest-and-digest response. At the core of this response is a survival mechanism; it is more important to deal with an immediate perceived danger or threat than to eat. The inhibition of appetite correlates with the duration and intensity of the stressor. Acute, intense stress inhibits feeding, while low-grade, chronic stress can increase appetite.

AgRP mRNA levels can be down-regulated following an acutely stressful event. This potential loss of AgRP function and consequent appetite-inhibition may contribute to the development of anorexia nervosa. High CRH levels are also involved in anorexia nervosa. Meanwhile, chronic stress stimulates the release of NPY, which increases appetite. However, NPY is associated with resilience and improved recovery

> Chronic stress stimulates the release of NPY, which increases appetite.

from post-traumatic stress disorder. Higher levels of Y1 and Y5 receptors in the amygdala and Y1 receptors in the forebrain result in reduced anxiety and fear response, allowing individuals to perform better under stressful conditions. NPY neurons also interact with dopaminergic reward and emotion pathways in the nucleus accumbens and amygdala respectively.

Nevertheless, higher NPY levels increase glucocorticoid levels in the blood, which stimulate gluconeogenesis, in turn causing a spike in blood glucose that activates insulin release. This chronic situation favours insulin resistance, resulting in high blood glucose levels and the risk of type 2 diabetes, as well as increased fat reserves. This effect is compounded as chronic stress continues to disrupt the HPA-axis function causing high circulating cortisol levels, which raise glucose and subsequently insulin levels, further increasing fat reserves, insulin resistance and hypertension. Hence the link between stress and cardiovascular disease, type 2 diabetes and obesity. High glucocorticoid levels continue to activate NPY release creating a vicious spiral. This spiral is confirmed by studies showing a significant reduction in obesity in rats following adrenalectomy.

Chronic stress during pregnancy can affect HPA regulation in offspring, most commonly causing a hyper-reactive HPA stress response, associated with behavioural disorders, attention deficits, schizophrenia, anxiety and depression. Chronic stress during pregnancy is also associated with slow language development and intellectual activity in offspring. If stress exposure is prolonged and extreme in early life, the above stress-related issues can be exacerbated. However, mild and infrequent stressors in early life can build stress resilience and enhance HPA function.

> The glucocorticoid excess created by stress increases feeding, weight and fat in an escalating cycle.

Therefore, the glucocorticoid excess created by stress increases feeding, weight and fat in an escalating cycle.

Glucocorticoids activate NPY release and modulate dopamine and serotonin release in the mesolimbic reward pathways to further increase the intake of highly palatable food.

Endogenous opioids and serotonin levels also play a key role in this chronic stress-induced eating. Exposure to rewarding stimuli reduces the stress response in the HPA and, therefore, chronic stress increases reward-seeking behaviour, such as eating highly palatable foods. We will look at this aspect later in the chapter.

Thus, we have seen in this section, that it is not the fight-or-flight, sudden, acute stress that usually triggers weight gain, in fact this stress reduces appetite and, if sufficiently intense, can influence the development of anorexia nervosa. Instead, it is the continual, low-grade, chronic psychosocial stress common to modern living that is an important contributing factor to weight gain and the development of obesity and eating disorders such as bulimia.

> The continual, low-grade, chronic psychosocial stress common to modern living is an important contributing factor to weight gain.

Subordinate individuals in the workplace have higher levels of cortisol, higher levels of NPY, greater leptin resistance, increased appetite and greater visceral body fat than dominant individuals. This neuroendocrine profile coupled with the ubiquitous availability of highly palatable foods makes effective weight management a difficult challenge for vast sections of the working population.

Self-soothing – The Edible Comfort Blanket
Eating may be a way of inducing the body back into rest-and-digest mode in the face of continuous stress. Stress intensifies the reward perception associated with food, thus increasing the psychological over physiological factors of eating.

Self-soothing is an aspect of emotional eating aimed at reducing stress and anxiety, as well as counteracting some of the emotional states listed previously, such as depression, loneliness, avoidance and helplessness. It is often known as comfort eating.

Certain foods, in particular sweet, fatty foods, such as ice-cream and chocolate, and highly palatable carbohydrates, such as pasta, chips and pizza, which are registered from childhood as treats or rewards, are those consumed most during bouts of comfort eating. The positive associations that have been created with these foods are a self-soothing method of counterbalancing or numbing negative emotions.

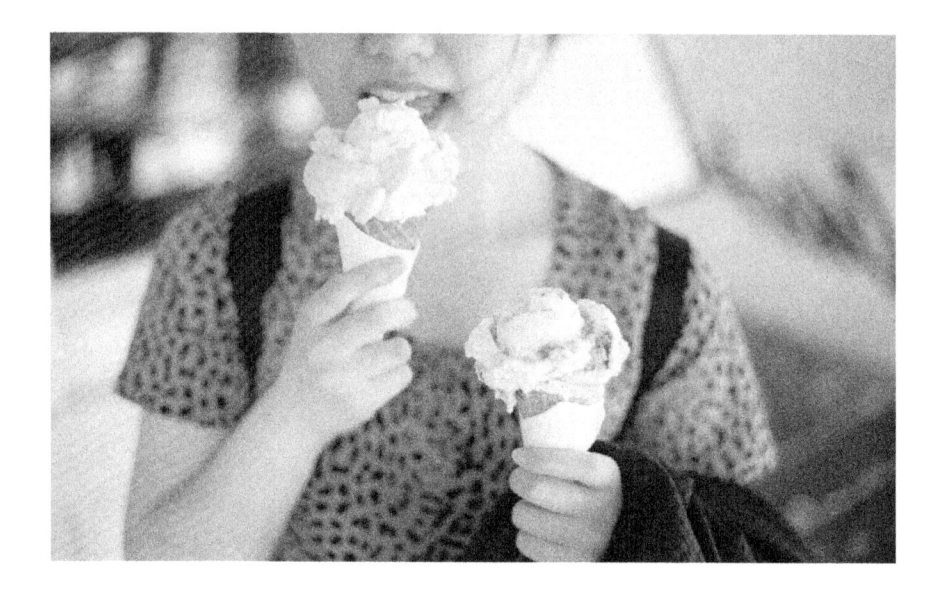

Deep-seated insecurities and social phobias can also increase the subconscious desire to create a physical barrier around the body in the form of layers of fat that insulate the individual from social interaction and intimacy.

Comfort eating can become an ingrained habit of self-soothing to allay fears, anxiety and negative emotions, such as sadness, loneliness, anger, low self-esteem and frustration. It can also function as a distraction from more pressing matters, worries or responsibilities or just to fill the hole of boredom. Psychologically there is a void, one of emptiness, helplessness, exhaustion, sadness or lovelessness, that comfort eating attempts to physically fill.

Self-soothing in the form of comfort eating is a goal-directed behaviour. If initiated in childhood where food was offered to make the child feel better regardless of hunger or physical requirements, or indeed to reward or celebrate events, then this behaviour can be a deeply ingrained, habitual response. As an adult, therefore, comfort eating will be a go-to emotional reaction, especially to negative emotions. This automatic response will have been encoded in the amygdala, with associated emotional memories, and in the dorsal striatum, which is in the basal ganglia of the brain and is a key component of the motor and reward systems.

The Reward System
The epicentre of the reward system lies adjacent to the dorsal striatum in the nucleus accumbens of the ventral striatum. The nucleus accumbens initiates goal-directed behaviour and, through repetition, it is reinforced in the dorsal striatum.

The reward system is responsible for the desire to consume (incentive salience) and positive reinforcement (associative learning) based on the effect of consumption, usually pleasurable. The reward system greatly conditions behaviour, it identifies the reward as an attractive motivation that stimulates its consumption.

The reward system is a survival mechanism that renders certain rewards, such as palatable food, sexual intercourse and parental investment, sufficiently pleasurable that we are stimulated to seek them out and engage in them.

> The reward system is a survival mechanism that renders certain rewards, such as palatable food, sexual intercourse and parental investment, sufficiently pleasurable that we are stimulated to seek them out and engage in them.

The reward system is predominantly dopaminergic. It includes the mesolimbic pathway, which connects the ventral tegmental area (VTA) in the midbrain to the nucleus accumbens and olfactory tubercle in the ventral striatum. The substantia nigra supplies dopamine to the striatum. The nucleus accumbens also receives input from the hippocampus, amygdala and medial prefrontal cortex and, when activated by these glutamatergic neurons, releases GABA onto the ventral pallidum, one of the brain's pleasure centres. The ventral pallidum also receives dopinaminergic inputs from the VTA, which allow it to mediate the perception of pleasure from certain stimuli, such as highly palatable foods.

Together this system of neurons regulates the value associated with an experience (prefrontal cortex), through memory associations (amygdala and hippocampus) and pleasure (VTA and ventral pallidum), as well as the motivational salience (nucleus accumbens), and then encodes the motor programs required to obtain the reward in the future (dorsal striatum). The greater the dopamine release, the greater will be the motivation to obtain the reward and the reinforcement of incentive salience (desire/wanting) for the reward in the future. This system clearly plays a pivotal role in the development and maintenance of addictive and compulsive behaviour.

Therefore, when the consumption of food, particularly highly palatable food, has become associated with reward through this dopamine reward system, the drive to eat is compulsive. Normally, the pre-frontal cortex is able to intervene by controlling the impulse to overeat, but stress or reduced serotonin levels can reduce its functionality. When the pre-frontal cortex does not intervene, the impulse is transformed from a goal-orientated habit to a compulsive stimulus-response habit mediated directly by the dorsal striatum. Activation of dopamine will reinforce the incentive salience to engage in the behaviour in the future. The more dopamine released by the reward, the greater the incentive salience. Dopamine polymorphisms, where the reward circuitry associated with food is absent, greatly increase the risk of developing anorexia nervosa.

> When the consumption of food, particularly highly palatable food, has become associated with reward through the dopamine reward system, the drive to eat is compulsive. Normally, the pre-frontal cortex is able to intervene by controlling the impulse to overeat, but stress or reduced serotonin levels can reduce its functionality.

CART (a satiety signal) is also released in response to repeated dopamine release in the nucleus accumbens and is thought to play a key role in the dopamine reward system. It has been seen to positively affect outcomes in alcohol withdrawal and cocaine addiction treatment. Reduced activity of CART is associated with depression, overeating, weight gain and susceptibility to drug addiction.

Ghrelin is also active in the dopamine reward system, increasing the tendency towards highly palatable or rewarding foods, such as pizza and ice cream, and drinks, such as alcohol. This hedonic consumption of food increases ghrelin levels, as well as dopamine levels, which may explain high levels of ghrelin in obese individuals, who ordinarily should have lower ghrelin levels than lean individuals.

The incentive salience of a reward is thus controlled by the dopamine reward system. However, the extent to which the reward is enjoyed is dependent upon the opioid system. Endogenous opioids include enkephalins, dynorphin and endorphins (processed from POMC), examples of exogenous opioids include morphine, heroin and nicotine.

Dopamine does not mediate the pleasure derived from the reward, which explains why drug addicts continue to want drugs even when the drugs no longer produce a euphoric reaction and also why compulsive eaters continue to eat excessive amounts of food even when the pleasure derived from the food diminishes.

Therefore, brain circuitry involved in compulsive eating is similar to that of drug addiction, also in the way in which it increases the reward threshold such that motivation requires an ever-greater reward, such as more and more food or drugs respectively, and the subject becomes less motivated to participate in other activities, such as physical exercise or social interaction. Also, negative consequences become insufficient deterrents to reward seeking.

Glucose reacts with the opioid system in the brain, making sugary and highly palatable foods more pleasurable to consume. Studies show that pain tolerance is significantly increased following sucrose ingestion. This analgesic effect is utilised for procedural pain in neonates; for example, a glucose solution may be administered prior to a heel prick. Studies found that binge eaters ate 22% less after administration with an opiate antagonist. Furthermore, recovering drug addicts going through opiate withdrawal experience intense cravings for glucose-rich foods and typically experience significant weight gain during their recovery period. Indirectly, consumption of energy-dense foods also increases the endogenous levels of endorphins in the brain, which trigger the pleasure centres. Furthermore, certain foods, such as chocolate, contain high levels of phenylethylamine, which regulates endorphin release.

The effect of endorphin release is particularly sought after to dampen stress as it gives an instantaneous sense of relaxation. Endorphins can alternatively be increased through exercise, positive social interaction and sleep, so a sedentary lifestyle coupled with lack of sleep and social isolation increases the propensity to activate opioid release through binge eating.

Thus, emotional eating is triggering dopamine and opioid reward circuits in the brain to counteract stress and negative emotions. In order to disengage from this form of compulsive overeating, alternative methods must be found to appease these reward circuits and counteract the triggering factors of stress and negative emotions on eating behaviour. We will now explore these alternative routes.

The Serotonin Connection
Serotonin is most commonly known as the body's happy neurotransmitter, responsible for feelings of joy and wellbeing. It is a mood regulator and anxiolytic (it inhibits the release of noradrenaline from adrenergic nerves), but it is also a powerful appetite suppressant and a sleep modulator (as a precursor to melatonin, the sleep hormone).

> Serotonin is the body's happy neurotransmitter, responsible for feelings of joy and wellbeing. It is a powerful appetite suppressant and a sleep.

Studies have shown that serotonin is upgraded by eating sugary or starchy carbohydrate-rich meals. Tryptophan, the building block of serotonin, finds it difficult to pass into the brain if it is competing with other amino acids, from a protein-rich meal, for example. However, a glucose-rich meal triggers insulin, which transports nutrients, including amino acids, into cells. Studies show that rats select carbohydrate-rich meals over protein-rich meals when their serotonin levels are low.

Tryptophan has a tendency to bind loosely with circulating albumin, which reduces its transportation into cells. For these reasons, competition between amino acids at the blood-brain barrier is reduced after a carbohydrate-rich meal and tryptophan passes through more easily and can get converted to serotonin, which reduces anxiety and appetite quickly.

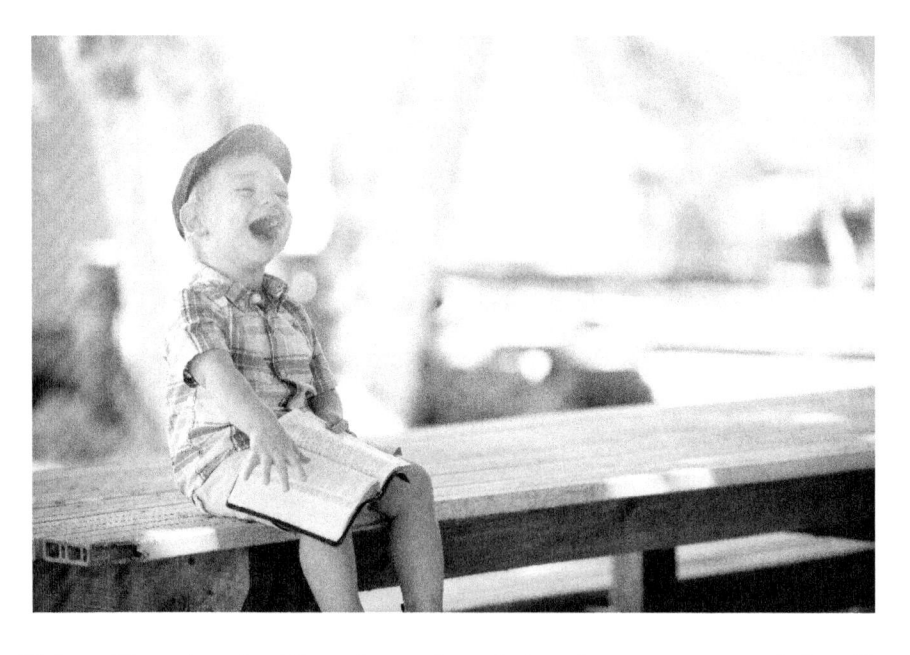

This effect is significantly reduced in the presence of insulin resistance, but it is greatly increased through exercise where plasma concentrations of branched chain amino acids (BCAAs – leucine, isoleucine and valine) are reduced and tryptophan levels are increased proportionately.

High levels of serotonin reduce appetite. Serotonin precursors, such as 5- Hydroxytryptophan (5-HTP), a supplement derived from the seeds of the Griffonia simplicifolia plant, have been found useful in controlling food cravings, especially carbohydrate cravings, and appetite, as well as, improving sleep and reducing stress. As we have seen, negative emotions, stress and poor sleep all contribute to excess eating, so serotonin is a powerful aid in weight management. Serotonin can be increased naturally by positive emotions, exposure to bright light, exercise and the use of supplements, such as 5-HTP.

Our increasingly sedentary lives, passed mainly indoors, dampen serotonin levels that previously, with more active lives spent outdoors, could be higher and correlated with lower levels of obesity. Depression, seasonal affective disorder (SAD), nicotine withdrawal and premenstrual syndrome (PMS) all correlate with carbohydrate cravings and weight gain, which may be more a result of the primary problem of low serotonin levels.

> Our increasingly sedentary lives, passed mainly indoors, dampen serotonin levels that previously, with more active lives passed outdoors, could be higher and correlated with lower levels of obesity.

Similarly, tyrosine, the precursor to the catecholamines dopamine, adrenaline and noradrenaline, can enhance catecholamine production and release in a variety of circumstances, to reduce appetite and cravings. Sufficient tyrosine in the diet can, therefore, also aid weight management.

The Leptin Connection
In addition to its effect on physiological satiety cues, leptin also influences psychological cues by its influence on the reward factor of eating. Leptin receptors are found in the limbic system and are highly expressed on dopaminergic neurons in the VTA, which we have seen project to the striatum, the amygdala and the prefrontal cortex.

High leptin levels correlate with a reduction in incentive salience associated with feeding, acting principally on the ventral striatum, but also via a combined effect of simultaneously inhibiting NPY/AgRP neurons and melanocyte stimulating hormone (MSH), thus modulating the mesolimbic dopamine signal and reducing food intake. Furthermore, the lateral hypothalamus contains a population of ObR-expressing neurons, which project directly to the ventral tegmental area. These leptin actions are opposed by antipsychotic drugs that act as dopamine receptor antagonists, which is probably why these drugs often cause weight gain as a side effect.

Leptin also acts in the nucleus accumbens of the ventral striatum affecting subjective measures of food liking. We usually seek highly palatable foods that are sweet or salty rather than bitter or sour. This information is conveyed by our sensory receptors and relayed to the thalamus and lateral frontal cerebral cortex, central nucleus of the amygdala and lateral hypothalamus area. Leptin deficiencies or leptin resistance increase the response to highly palatable foods, whereas high levels of leptin, reduce food liking ratings and consequently reduce the salience or reward associated with feeding.

Counteracting leptin's effects, ghrelin also regulates feeding through the mesolimbic system, by stimulating dopamine neurons in the VTA and promoting dopamine turnover in the nucleus accumbens of the ventral striatum. This added reward incentive aspect of physiological cues of appetite encourages excessive eating beyond satiety, which allows energy storage for times of scarcity. However, in times of constant availability of highly palatable foods, this mechanism encourages excessive weight gain and obesity.

The ability of leptin to reduce appetite and compulsive eating is impaired by stress and depression, both of which down-regulate leptin production. In fact, depression has been linked to both leptin deficiency and leptin resistance. Obese individuals have high leptin levels, but also have high leptin resistance, and they have been shown to be 20% more likely to suffer from depression than non-obese individuals. Leptin receptors are widely distributed in the brain, which immediately indicates a broader function than just energy homeostasis. In particular, the leptin receptor is highly expressed in the hippocampus, cortex and amygdala, brain areas involved in mood regulation.

> The ability of leptin to reduce appetite and compulsive eating is impaired by stress and depression, both of which down-regulate leptin production.

Furthermore, with respect to depression, leptin enhances mesolimbic dopamine activity and may modulate the serotonin system, with a high proportion of serotonin neurons expressing the leptin receptor. It also, as mentioned earlier, modulates HPA function, down-regulating ACTH and CRH release, thus attenuating the stress response. It also acts directly on the adrenal gland, inhibiting basal and ACTH-stimulated cortisol release.

The Role of Oxytocin
We have seen how leptin and several monoamine neurotransmitters are important in regulating the HPA axis, especially dopamine, serotonin and noradrenaline. There is also evidence that an increase in oxytocin, resulting, for instance, from positive social interaction, acts to suppress the HPA axis and thereby counteracts stress, depression and reduces stress-fuelled overeating.

Particularly known for its role in maternal bonding, orgasm and couple bonding, this neuropeptide, produced by the PVN of the hypothalamus and released from the pituitary gland (oxytocin receptor-expressing cells are also located in the amygdala and in the bed nucleus of the stria terminalis), evokes feelings of complete contentment, calmness, security and love. It is, therefore, anathema to feelings of anxiety, fear and stress, as well as hunger, especially compulsive hunger. Therefore, social support, positive social

> Social support, positive social interaction and intimacy can be effective methods for counteracting stress, depression and compulsive eating.

interaction and intimacy can be effective methods for counteracting stress, depression and compulsive eating.

Oxytocin requires vitamin C as an essential vitamin cofactor in its synthesis. In fact, increased vitamin C administration was found to increase the production of oxytocin in ovarian tissue. Meanwhile, the oxytocin receptor is a G-protein-coupled receptor, which requires magnesium and cholesterol to function effectively.

The Psychology of Deprivation
The standard approach to instigating weight loss in cases of unhealthy weight gain or obesity is to restrict a subject's food intake. This is usually prescribed by a doctor or self-imposed. In either case, the diet is one of restriction and the aim is weight loss. How the brain formulates these two parameters, that is, the concepts of restriction or deprivation and loss, is key to the potential success or failure of the programme.

Restriction and loss do not have an affinity with the reward system and the inborn drive for pleasure. Previously in this chapter, we saw how our physiological cues of hunger and satiety seem designed to more strongly avert starvation than they are to prevent excessive food intake, so the body will work against restriction by regulating hunger cues accordingly, downgrading our basal metabolic rate and interpreting caloric restriction as a stressor. These are evolutionary survival mechanisms that have ensured our continued presence on this planet.

It is clear that given the strength and intelligence of our body, we need to reframe the paradigm of healthy weight management in such a way that all elements involved are positive and on the same team.

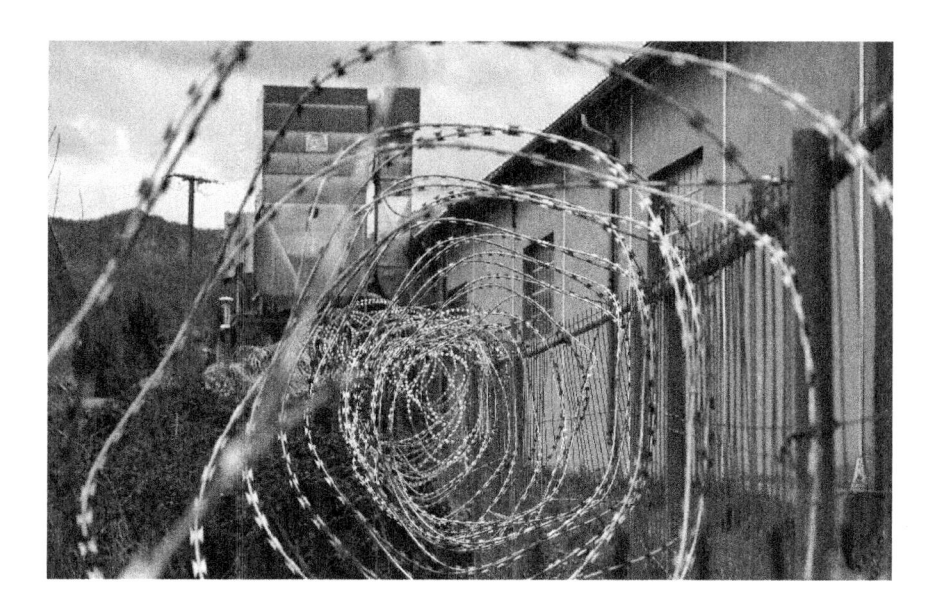

We need to redefine the context from being a fight between our desire and our will into being a team effort in which each factor contributes to moving in the same intended direction. This new context is principally framed within the mind and this chapter is an acknowledgement of the vast importance of psychology in successful weight management.

The psychological effects of restrictive diets are well known. One famous study by Dr. Ancel Keys at the University of Minnesota was carried out on conscientious objectors during World War II. Thirty-six healthy young men were put on a calorie-restricted diet for a year and required to walk twenty-two miles a week. The aim was not to tackle obesity, which wasn't yet a widespread problem, but rather to understand how best to refeed a population that may have been living in starvation.

Their daily food allowance was around 1600 calories, half their consumption prior to starting the study, and it was modified weekly to achieve weight loss of about 2.5lbs (1.1kg) a week. The effects of this regime included lethargy, irritability, anxiety, dizziness, cold intolerance, inability to concentrate, reduced coordination, reduced libido, muscle soreness, hair loss, food obsession, depression and there was also one case of self-mutilation and suicidal tendencies.

After the experiment ended, the men binged and gained substantial weight. Despite the above results and the on-going struggle overweight patients have with traditional dieting, caloric restriction is still the method prescribed by most doctors today for weight loss.

> A restrictive diet followed by a bout of binge eating is a very familiar cycle for many people struggling to achieve weight loss.

A restrictive diet followed by a bout of binge eating is a very familiar cycle for many people struggling to achieve weight loss. The deprivation leads to an obsessive focus on food and weight and the frustration builds up until it can no longer be withstood and the dieter binges on all those foods that were prohibited during the diet. This yo-yo effect often sets the dieter up for a lifelong struggle as successive restrictive diets keep lowering the basal metabolic rate and render it more and more difficult to lose weight.

To the above context, we must add the damaging effects on self-esteem of repeated failure to meet a weight loss goal, as well as failure to comply with an internalised, unrealistic societal standard of body size and success.

Apart from the metabolic adaptation to restrictive diets, which we will study in more detail in Chapter Three, there is the restrictive paradigm, the notion of loss, weight watching and often self-flagellation that runs against the reward circuitry of the brain, which instead seeks pleasure. Often an externally imposed regime is only sustainable if we fully appropriate it as our own intention and it will only work long-term if we are able to rewire our reward systems to support the goal rather than thwart it.

The reframing process may need to start in the language we use; the concept of "losing" weight is counterintuitive to reward behaviour. A loss sounds like a failure and a punishment. We can replace use of the term "losing" weight with releasing, unloading, discharging, freeing excess fat or achieving or reaching a healthy weight and a stronger, healthier body. The choice of reward-associated food need not be unhealthy, but can be both nutritious and delicious.

> The reframing process may need to start in the language we use; the concept of "losing" weight is counterintuitive to reward behaviour. A loss sounds like a failure and a punishment.

Understanding that emotional eating is also a method used to soothe or numb negative emotions, presupposes the need to find alternative tools to acknowledge and cope with negative emotions to replace the emotional eating that deregulates weight management. We list some techniques at the end of this chapter to replace emotional eating with healthier habits.

Body positivity, appreciation and acceptance of body shape in the present moment can also reverse some of the negative emotions that lead to emotional eating. Focusing on the health of the body, the fact that it supports life, appreciation of all the activities the body allows us to enjoy, helps us to reframe our use of food as a means to best nourish and care for the body instead of as a punishing restrictive framework that is periodically violated.

As we will learn in Chapter Four, physical exercise as a means of tipping the energy equation in favour of weight loss is not always a fool-proof method of weight management. However, psychologically, physical exercise has positive effects on mood and, if we can find a form of physical exercise that we really enjoy, it is a pleasurable, sustainable and healthy habit that will reinforce a positive body image and reduce emotional eating.

Eating Disorders
While we will not analyse eating disorders in great detail, it is important in the scope of this book to study certain characteristics that shift weight management into deregulated appetite and weight issues.

Anorexia Nervosa
Anorexia is characterised by extreme limitation of food intake and an intense fear of being fat. Ghrelin levels are high and leptin levels low, but the individual represses the urge to eat. Studies show that reward and motivation circuits are not engaged in the brains of anorexic individuals. Instead, self-control circuitry is activated, which in itself may represent a reward, the achievement of resisting temptation and avoiding weight gain.

Psychological causes of anorexia may be similar to those involved in other eating disorders, such as low self-esteem, depression, anxiety, loneliness or a sense of no control over one's life, but the outcome is severe weight loss and the risk of death. Cases of anorexia nervosa have increased in the last century, especially in cultures or professions in which there is a strong social pressure to be thin, such as dance, fashion and gymnastics, but also in countries in which the media presents limited body ideals that do not represent the full range of healthy body shapes. Popularity, desirability and happiness are continuously linked to thinness rather than health through social media, which compounds the prevalence of this eating disorder.

> Anorexia deregulates the serotonin system, which heightens the obsessiveness and anxiety characteristic of anorexia.

Anorexia deregulates the serotonin system, principally

through tryptophan depletion (a precursor of serotonin), which heightens the obsessiveness and anxiety characteristic of anorexia. Anorexics also show extreme cognitive control regarding eating behaviour, which is associated with alterations in the dorsal anterior cingulate cortex.

Binge Eating Disorder and Bulimia Nervosa
Binge eating disorder is characterised by excessive, often uncontrollable, bouts of eating. Bulimia is characterised by the same bouts of excessive eating, but is usually followed by purging by self-induced vomiting, extreme physical exercise or the use of laxatives. Both disorders, like anorexia, are characterised by an excessive preoccupation with physical appearance and body weight, as well as a distortion of body image.

As with anorexia, binge eaters and bulimics often suffer from low self-esteem, anxiety and depression. These disorders are most prevalent among young women. Media bombardment of idealised thin bodies can cause young women to compare themselves unfavourably to the media model of beauty. This self-objectification can lead to body dissatisfaction, low self-esteem and eating disorders.

Aside from social pressure, these eating disorders are an extreme form of emotional eating and have been correlated with negative emotions of loneliness and social isolation, as well as with stress, anxiety or memories of child abuse. It has been shown that certain parenting techniques, particularly coercing children to eat beyond satiety or using food to reward or otherwise influence behaviour, can lead to an unhealthy relationship with food and facilitate obesity and eating disorders.

As in the case of anorexia, binge eating and bulimia can cause a deregulation of the HPA axis, which throws off-balance the production of neurotransmitters, neuropeptides and hormones. Elevated levels of homocysteine are found in individuals with eating disorders as well as low levels of serotonin and serotenergic responsiveness, as are also common in individuals with depression.

Gut Health

Individuals with eating disorders generally have poor gut health and, in particular, elevated levels of autoantibodies that affect the hormones and neuropeptides that regulate appetite and the stress response.

> Individuals with eating disorders generally have poor gut health and, in particular, elevated levels of autoantibodies that affect the hormones and neuropeptides that regulate appetite and the stress response.

The gut-brain axis is regulated by gut microbiota (gut bacteria). This complex system not only regulates gastrointestinal function, but also has an effect on mood, cognitive function and stress resilience. Stress can alter the microbiota profile and, vice-versa, an alteration in the microbiota caused by a change in diet, overeating or eating disorders can deregulate the HPA axis and influence stress responsiveness.

The gut microbiota also affects the structure and function of the amygdala, which we have seen plays a vital role in emotional learning and identification of potential stressors that trigger the stress response.

95% of serotonin in the body is produced in the gut and regulates gastrointestinal secretion, motility and pain perception. As we have seen, it is also heavily implicated in weight management. Brain serotonin influences mood, cognition and appetite. Dysfunctional serotonin signalling is implicated in both mood and gut issues and suggests a high level of co-morbidity between the two. Gut microbiota is also key in tryptophan availability and metabolism, which regulates serotonin levels.

Improvements in gut microbiota, and consequently reductions in stress-related behaviour and HPA activation, have been shown with the use of prebiotics (non-digestible fibre), probiotics and omega-3 fatty acids.

The Set Point

Let us turn now to the elusive concept of set point. The physiological cues of appetite studied earlier in this chapter are regulated around a set point of energy homeostasis or balance, just as room temperature is by a thermostat. The body manages hunger and satiety signals so that weight remains stable around a particular level. But how does the body determine this set point and can it be changed? If so, by what methods can the set point be reprogramed to a healthier level?

Generally, we can have wide fluctuations in food intake and physical exercise, but our weight tends to remain within a fairly narrow range. We have seen that the body defends against weight loss more than it does against weight gain, but, if the regulatory endogenous energy thermostat is functioning correctly and is not overridden, fluctuations in food intake and physical exercise will be modified to always keep the body at a set weight. What determines this set point? It is rooted in physiology, genetics and molecular biology, but also in psychology.

> We can have wide fluctuations in food intake and physical exercise, but our weight tends to remain within a fairly narrow range. This set point is rooted in physiology, genetics and molecular biology, but also in psychology.

What happens when this physiological system that has evolved in an environment of variable food availability gets transplanted to an obesogenic environment of constant food availability? We have seen how the reward system ensures that we take advantage of the presence of energy-dense foods, but does the set point enforce a regulatory limit on eating too? It can only do so where the patterns of emotional eating have not yet deregulated the physiological system, causing insulin and leptin resistance and imbalances of the HPA-axis. These conditions set up an escalation of weight gain.

The set point is maintained by physiological cues, it is determined by genetic cues, but its blueprint may be established and maintained by the image of ourselves we carry in our minds. Here, we leave the world of thermodynamics and enter the world of quantum physics to consider the mind-body connection.

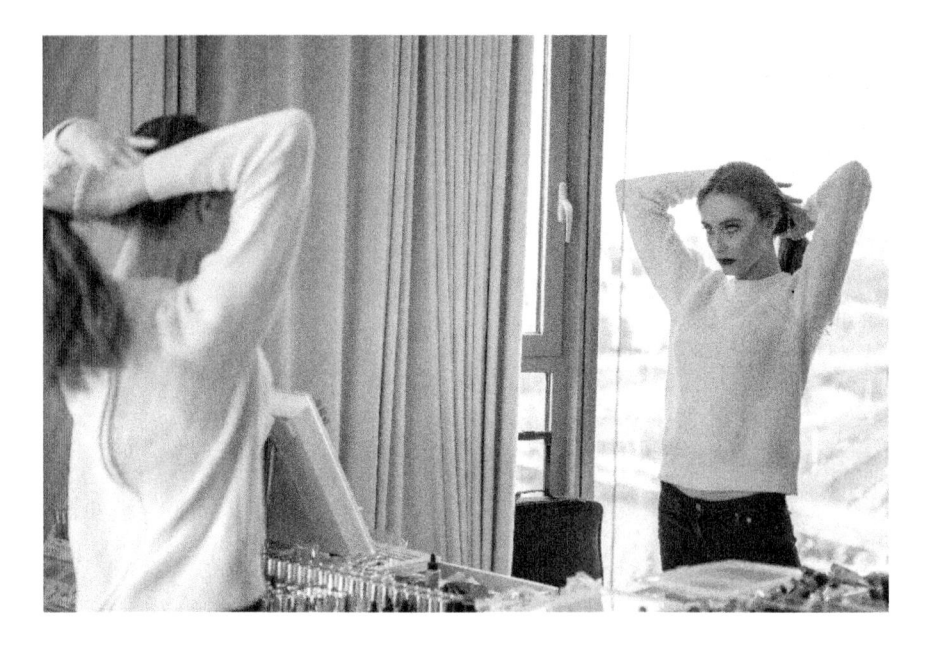

Does our body shape conform to what we imagine it to be? Clearly not in the case of body dysmorphia, but otherwise does the image we hold of ourselves also act as a thermostat to curb excessive weight gain or loss? If the internalised image we have of ourselves is overweight, will we sabotage our efforts to lose weight such that our physical bodies conform to the mental picture we have of ourselves? Is it necessary to reprogram this internal blueprint for any weight change to be maintained? Studies have shown that a positive body image improves weight management and enhances the results of a weight loss programme based on dietary modifications and increased physical exercise. By holding a favourable image in our mind of our physical appearance, it can act as a new thermostat reading upon which to recalibrate our weight.

> By holding a favourable image in our mind of our physical appearance, it can act as a new thermostat reading upon which to recalibrate our weight.

Mindful Eating
The first step in reducing excessive eating is to understand its root cause. As a highly addictive behaviour, emotional eating is often an automatic circuit, that is, the individual consumes excessive quantities of food without conscious intent, but instead as a subconscious reaction to a variety of triggers. This can happen most easily when eating is combined with an activity such as watching television or surfing the internet.

Mindful eating means being fully present in the action of eating, giving our exclusive attention to what we are eating and nothing else. This technique will be difficult at first to those who use eating as a means to escape from negative emotions. However, it can have numerous health benefits.

When we become fully aware of what we are doing, our focus allows us to take in more details about the action. In the case of eating, we notice what we are eating, how we prepared it, the smell, the texture, the taste, the colours. We slow down, spend more time savouring the food and chewing fully, instead of shovelling food down while our attention is elsewhere.

Mindful eating allows us to fully reap the reward and pleasure aspects of eating (dopamine and opioid circuitry). It also allows time for our satiety signals to register before we have already eaten excessively. Finally, it facilitates digestion and gastrointestinal health by sufficient chewing and by creating a relaxed window in which the body will not be distracted, stressed or over-excited by inputs from the television or the computer.

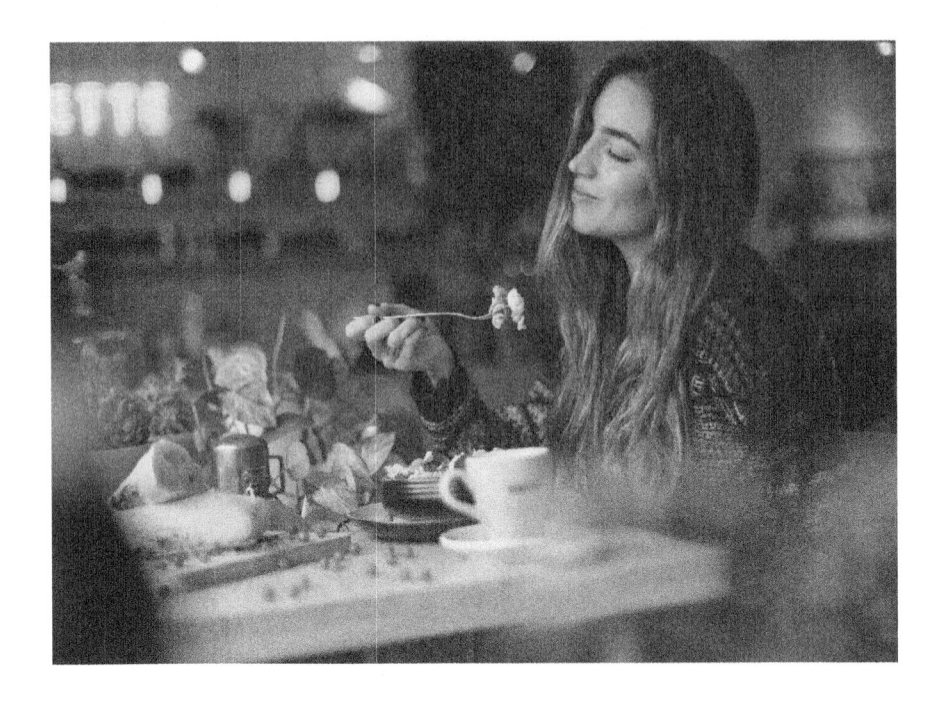

Mindful eating practices can uncover the thought processes that trigger compulsive eating and have been successful in reducing episodes of binge eating in individuals with binge-eating disorder and bulimia nervosa.

Cognitive Behavioural Therapy
Mindful eating will make it easier to identify the triggers to overeating. Cognitive behavioural therapy (CBT) teaches that an individual's reaction to external stimuli is based upon their own perception, perspective and thoughts regarding any trigger and not dependent on the trigger itself in many instances. As such, we have the freedom to change thought processes and thus change our reaction to any trigger.

CBT takes control upstream; from control over what we eat to control over what we are thinking, which may be driving food choices. It questions how thoughts regarding a situation may be triggering the negative emotions that are triggering emotional eating. Thoughts that generate positive emotions are less likely to drive the self-soothing of emotional comfort eating.

> CBT takes control upstream; from control over what we eat to control over what we are thinking, which may be driving food choices.

CBT involves reframing (seeing the stressful situation from different perspectives, distancing and detaching from our role in the drama), learning to set limits and boundaries, learning to relish a challenge and planning ways within our control to overcome a situation. Journaling can be a useful technique in identifying and articulating the emotions that usually spark emotional eating.

Relaxation Techniques
Any technique that counteracts chronic stress and anxiety will reduce emotional eating. Generally, the most effective techniques cause us to slow down (decelerating our automatic drive into emotional eating) or divert (derailing the propulsion energy away from emotional eating and into a healthier activity). We must all find a technique or a variety of techniques that can counteract the stress response in every situation and reduce chronic stress in our daily lives. Not every method will work for everyone; the best activities to choose are those that create the greatest sense of pleasure and peace for you. Examples may include massage, yoga, dance, music, art, breathing techniques, a warm bath or a walk in nature.

Modern life bombards us with sensory inputs. We live connected to technology. Many researchers have seen a link between rising obesity rates and the technology explosion. Internet and smartphones have allowed work and communication to reach us everywhere and all the time; we are constantly available to others and rarely disconnect from technology or switch off altogether for any significant length of time. This cognitive overload increases emotional eating as a subconscious escape tactic. Technology also disrupts sleep. Sleep deprivation is associated with an increased risk of overeating and obesity. We must all, therefore, learn to set boundaries on our use of technology to create digital-free spaces in time that are conducive to deep relaxation.

Another relaxation technique that increases the release of serotonin, oxytocin and endorphins, reducing the pull of emotional eating, is positive social interaction. Studies have shown that individuals who cultivate loving, satisfying relationships are happier, have fewer health problems and live longer.

> Studies have shown that individuals who cultivate loving, satisfying relationships are happier, have fewer health problems and live longer.

Self-Esteem
Low self-esteem is built on the negative beliefs we have constructed about ourselves. They may have been passed on by our parents or caregivers in the form of negative criticism when we were children, or from others in the form of teasing or bullying, but at some point they have become so internalised that they have solidified into beliefs we hold about ourselves. This internal critic is a constant reminder that we are too much of one thing and not enough of another and it undermines our confidence, our happiness, our contentment and our self-esteem. Emotional eating may be a means of escaping this voice or punishing or comforting ourselves for not measuring up to its demands.

A shift to kindness and compassion towards ourselves improves our relationship not only with ourselves but also with others. Shifting from inner critic to inner mentor or friend, encouraging and nurturing, can bolster self-esteem and transform negative into positive emotions. This shift paves the way for self-acceptance and greater self-understanding. Understanding our own needs, acknowledging them and ensuring that we take care of ourselves will render us happier and more capable of helping others and less likely to seek comfort or escape in food. One tool involves learning to befriend ourselves fully and to monitor our inner dialogue: do we speak to ourselves as we would to a beloved friend? Nurturing, appreciative and encouraging words counter the self-flagellation common to low self-esteem.

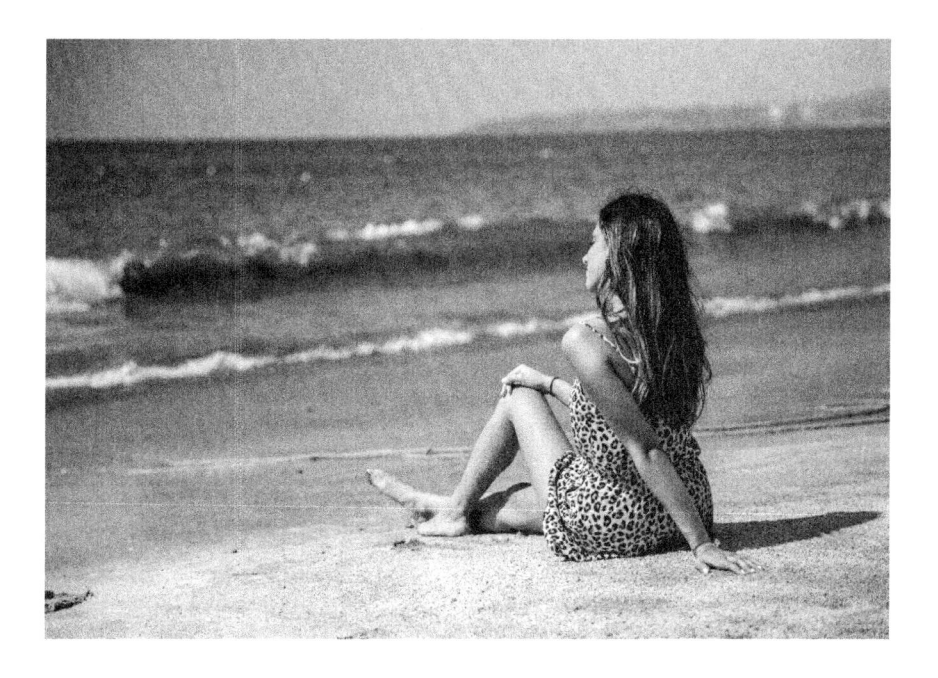

Self-esteem increases self-acceptance. By replacing the inner critic with a more nurturing voice, the heavy burden of self-judgment, guilt and shame is lifted. Similarly, we can dissolve the anger, frustration and resentment associated with blame and victimhood by taking responsibility for our own reactions to situations and other people's actions. Forgiveness of ourselves and others is a form of liberation and release, it ends punishment and is a self-soothing action that does not involve food intake. We accept that which we cannot change about ourselves and focus on our positive aspects and the ways in which we can develop and celebrate those aspects. This reduces the need for food as a way to numb uncomfortable feelings.

Being overweight in a society that values thinness carries with it a lot of stigma. The general view is that excessive weight shows a lack of self-discipline and gluttony. Self-acceptance and self-esteem are key tools in surviving the damaging effects of such stigma. Self-esteem increases self-care; we learn to look after ourselves better. We tend towards healthier choices, such as a more nutritious diet, more physical exercise, more rest and relaxation. This increases appreciation for the body and its health over derogatory comparisons with cultural ideals.

> Self-esteem increases self-care; we learn to look after ourselves better. We tend towards healthier choices, such as a more nutritious diet, more physical exercise, more rest and relaxation.

We can also learn to foster a sense of gratitude for the body. We can favour appreciation of the body's abilities rather than focusing solely on perceived flaws. This approach promotes better food choices and reduces the incidence of binges. We can choose to approach food as a way of looking after the body by providing the best nourishment possible rather than seeking temporary pleasure or punishment of the body with poor food choices.

We have seen previously that an influx of positive emotions satisfies the reward circuits of the brain, leads to higher levels of serotonin, dopamine and endogenous opioids, counterbalances chronic stress and reduces appetite and our tendency to overeat. Self-esteem that presupposes a new love and appreciation towards oneself fulfils these requirements.

New Rewards

In order to replace highly palatable food as a motivating reward, an equally motivating alternative must be found. We must shift our perspective from weight watching to a more compelling purpose.

Emotional eating is fuelled by stress, depression, avoidance, sadness, exhaustion and frustration, but a new positive focus or healthy obsession can avert the automatic compulsion to eat. Finding an overriding purpose or goal in life can take the focus off food, whether it is overeating or dieting. A new, exciting purpose can supplant constant weight-watching or food cravings as the top priority.

> Finding an overriding purpose or goal in life can take the focus off food, whether it is overeating or dieting. A new, exciting purpose can supplant constant weight-watching or food cravings as the top priority.

Individuals who have successfully lost weight and kept it off exhibit cognitive control when presented with food cues. They have retrained their responses. Unsuccessful dieters continue to respond addictively to food cues. Studies have shown that for those most prone to emotional eating, the mere sight or thought of food can produce high levels of insulin in anticipation of intake. New rewards upon which to focus will diminish the obsessive lure of the buffet. The power can be taken out of the stimulus by reconditioning priorities.

The focus on weight loss goals, dieting and weight-watching can become all-consuming. Having goals and activities that eclipse an obsessive relationship with food has been proven to be more effective for weight management than another diet, as it presupposes a more intuitive approach to eating that is more in tune with the

> The focus on weight loss goals, dieting and weight-watching can become all-consuming. Having goals and activities that eclipse an obsessive relationship with food has been proven to be more effective for weight management than another diet.

body's physiological cues and real needs as opposed to its psychological triggers.

A focus on prioritising optimum health over weight loss goals is also a more successful approach. An interest in good nutrition or fitness can help. As well as the physical benefits, adherence to regular physical exercise has psychological benefits. As mentioned previously, exercise releases endorphins, which reduce the urge to eat compulsively. Exercise alleviates mood disorders and depression, it attenuates stress, builds emotional resilience and increases levels of happiness. The choice of sport is less important than the assiduity and enjoyment of participation.

Understanding Mindset
We have seen how the body has a tightly regulated system that controls energy balance such that energy intake is matched to energy expenditure and weight is maintained around an internal set point, much like a thermostat regulates room temperature. The brain receives several signals from the gastrointestinal tract and the pancreas regarding energy intake and from the periphery regarding energy reserves and regulates hunger and satiety signals accordingly.

When this orchestra of neurotransmitter and endocrine signals is working in symphony, appetite effectively regulates body weight around a set level. Any excess in food intake is balanced with a subsequent fall in food intake regulated by satiety signals to return energy balance to the same level as before and vice versa, a fall in food intake increases hunger signals to restore energy balance by increasing food intake. This is why it is so difficult to change weight from the body's internal set point; the body fights through powerful hunger/satiety signals to restore balance.

However, we have seen that when these signals are ignored, when we habitually eat in the absence of hunger and when we out-eat our satiety, the finely tuned symphony is knocked off balance and can spiral out of control. Leptin resistance, as one example, creates escalating hunger signals that increase food intake, despite plentiful fat reserves, and leads to obesity.

The key is not to increase one satiety signal in order to counteract out-of-balance hunger signalling, but instead to restore balance to the whole system, so that each player has its time on stage bringing harmony and, above all, efficiency to the whole, in terms of weight management. As we have seen, each player delivers direct and collateral benefits that work in symphony. Much research has looked into knocking out the effects of certain signals, but, despite the effect on weight loss being achieved, the result is a diminished orchestra and an unstable new balance.

> The key is not to increase one satiety signal in order to counteract out-of-balance hunger signalling, but instead to restore balance to the whole system, so that each player has its time on stage bringing harmony and, above all, efficacy to the whole.

Together all these neuropeptides and hormones can greatly facilitate balanced, healthy weight management. However, when knocked out of balance, they can be precipitating factors in our failure to stabilise weight. Instead of fighting against the body's appetite and flagging energy levels, we will implement tools that harness the body's tendency towards easy and healthy weight management in harmonic and sustainable balance.

When eating becomes an automatic response ingrained in the reward circuitry of the brain, unmediated by conscious cognitive control, physiological cues of satiety go unheeded as the brain seeks the reward and pleasure associated with certain highly palatable foods. This addictive behaviour creates a preoccupation with food, involving cravings and seeking out food at the expense of engaging in other activities.

The addictive aspects of overeating require conscious attention and the application of certain techniques in order to help us retrain our automatic responses to environmental or emotional cues to eat. Therefore, an important step in weight management is self-awareness and mindfulness.

Cognitive Behavioural Therapy helps reframe our reactions to stressful or emotional stimuli. Visualisation techniques help reprogram the internalised image we hold of ourselves from overweight to healthy. If our internalised self-image remains overweight or obese, we are more likely to sabotage our own efforts to establish a stable, healthy weight, as the new external image will no longer be coherent with the mind's blueprint.

> The emotional nature of compulsive eating requires a kind and compassionate approach; self-flagellation worsens the issue.

The emotional nature of compulsive eating requires a kind and compassionate approach; self-flagellation worsens the issue. Devising and learning to seek new, healthier rewards is a process that requires repeated implementation to become a habit, which is why compassion is an essential component. Ingrained triggers can take time to substitute with healthier alternatives. Mindfulness and a kinder attitude to self will render the journey easier and smoother.

Healthier rituals will eventually supplant the habit of compulsive eating, which usually involves hunting down the most palatable foods followed by their excessive consumption. In contrast, mindful eating requires us to set aside time to eat, to slow down and to refrain from eating in conjunction with other activities, such as reading emails, watching television, scrolling through social media or surfing the internet. This approach also reduces the constant grazing that increases the risk of obesity.

We have seen that chronic stress not only disrupts physiological cues but also escalates emotional eating, which deregulates weight management causing obesity that further drives emotional eating in a vicious cycle. Integrating any form of stress reduction into our day will improve weight management. What constitutes stress reduction will differ from individual to individual, but could include activities such as yoga, meditation, exercise, meeting up with friends, having a massage, taking a warm bath, reading a book or watching a comedy.

MINDSET PROTOCOL
Considering what we have learnt in this chapter, the healthiest plan, most conducive to weight loss and management, is one that manages and balances both the physiological **and** the psychological cues to eat.

Step One: Stress Relief
As we learnt in this chapter, stress is a powerful driver of overeating through both physiological hunger cues and emotional hunger cues. We need to address stress in our lives, find ways of reducing stress (this may involve, for example, the need to change jobs or move to a safer area) and, because it can be difficult to eliminate stress completely, we need to balance any stress in our lives with an equal daily dose of relaxation.

Each of us has different preferences when it comes to how to relax, but the following list can provide inspiration for finding the best activities for balancing stress:
- ✓ A warm bath;
- ✓ A yoga session;
- ✓ Drawing or painting;
- ✓ Meditation;
- ✓ A walk in nature;
- ✓ A massage;
- ✓ A feel-good film or television series;
- ✓ Reading a book;
- ✓ Listening to relaxing music;
- ✓ Taking a nap;
- ✓ Meeting up with friends;
- ✓ Swimming in the sea;
- ✓ Dancing.

Step Two: Dietary Considerations

We will study nutrition in more detail in Chapter Three, but for now let's consider the following tips:
- ✓ Protein reduces ghrelin levels and so reduces hunger signals more than fat or carbohydrates. Try to integrate a good source of protein into every meal.
- ✓ Fat increases CCK levels that increase satiety. Try to integrate a good source of fat into every meal.
- ✓ Adiponectin breaks down fat reserves. The following botanicals promote the action of adiponectin: curcumin in turmeric, capsaicin in chilli peppers and cayenne pepper, gingerol in ginger and catechins in green tea. Try to integrate these into your daily diet.
- ✓ Vitamin C is essential for the production of oxytocin, the feel-good hormone that is so powerful for counterbalancing stress. Good sources of vitamin C include citrus fruits, berries, broccoli, peas and cauliflower.
- ✓ Ghrelin levels are higher in people with a vitamin D deficiency. Make sure you have sufficient vitamin D by

getting around 15 minutes exposure to sunlight every day and/or eating fatty fish, like mackerel or salmon. A vitamin D3 supplement is also a good option.
- ✓ Keep serotonin levels high through exposure to sunlight, physical exercise, positive social interaction and by supplementing with 5-HTP, a serotonin precursor, which has been found to reduce appetite and food cravings.

Step Three: Mindfulness
Being consciously aware of our thoughts and actions gives us greater influence over them. This entails slowing down and questioning our emotions. Getting a handle on how we feel and why we feel a certain way creates a conscious space that otherwise may just get automatically filled with food. It also creates a greater consideration for ourselves that invites a greater care and nourishment of our inner life. In this step, you can start a journaling practice, as well as introducing the following practices:
- ✓ When you eat, do not engage in any other activity. Focus solely on what you are eating; savour the colours, the texture, the smell and the flavours. Practice gratitude and appreciation for the food you eat and for the nourishment it provides.
- ✓ Express complete acceptance, appreciation and gratitude for your body, for all the ways in which it facilitates and supports your experience of life.
- ✓ Accept any ways in which you may not have made the best choice for yourself. Each breath is a new opportunity to make a better choice. Forgive yourself and let any condemning thoughts drift away.
- ✓ Shift your inner dialogue from inner critic to inner friend or mentor. Be kind and compassionate with yourself as you would be to your dearest friend. Encourage and nurture yourself.

Step Four: Your Set Point
The image you hold of yourself in your mind acts as a subconscious blueprint that the body replicates. If we see ourselves as overweight,

we are more likely to subconsciously sabotage our efforts to establish a new healthy weight. Readjust this image of yourself in order to give your body a new blueprint, a new set point of balance, by doing the following every day:

- ✓ Visualise yourself feeling happy and confident. Imagine yourself walking along a beach, feel the warmth of the sun on your skin, the freshness of the water on your feet, a light breeze caressing your skin. Notice how comfortable and relaxed you feel in your skin. Your body feels strong, healthy and full of energy. This is you.
- ✓ Find a photo of yourself at a time when your weight was your healthiest, when you felt fit and strong, happy and confident. Display this photo somewhere you will see it and look at it every day, perhaps on your fridge door. Relive how you felt in this body. This is you.

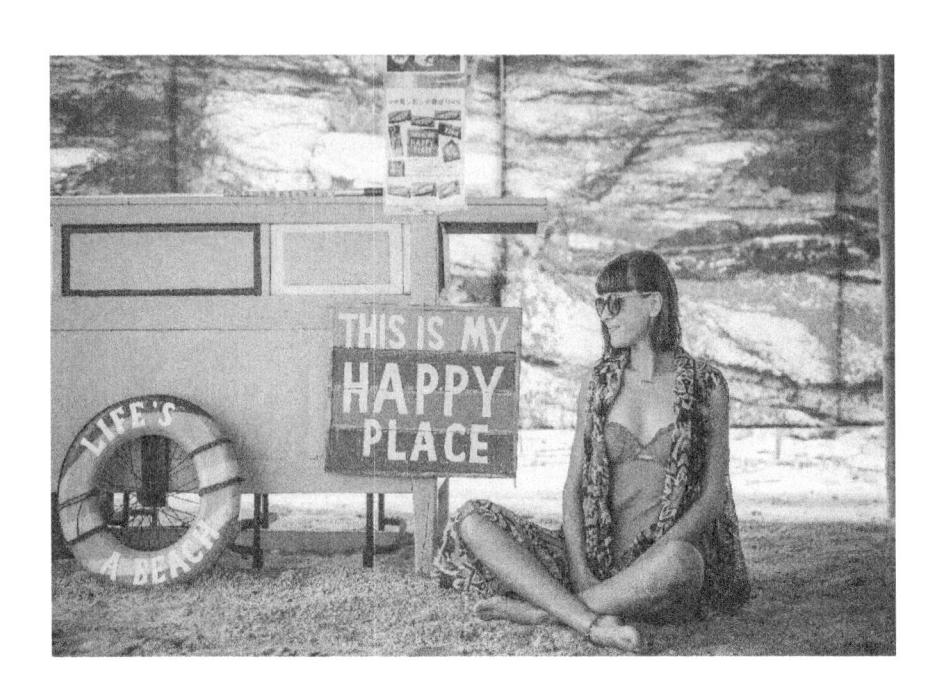

Step Five: New Goals
Once we accept ourselves fully, make friends with ourselves and learn to give ourselves the best care, we are ready to shift our focus from dieting and weight loss to a new compelling interest, hobby or purpose for our lives. We can ask ourselves the following questions to uncover our joy:

- ✓ What do I love doing? How can I make more space for that in my day?
- ✓ What music uplifts my mood and gives me energy?
- ✓ What unique gifts or talents do I have that I could enjoy and develop?
- ✓ How could I bring more joy to myself and others?
- ✓ How can I be of service to my family, my community, the world?

Allow time each day to daydream, prompted by the above questions. The busyness of our lives often immerses us, monopolises our thought processes and does not allow the room and serenity needed for new, inspiring ideas.

The above protocol addresses why we eat and promises to rebalance the body's physiological and psychological cues, allowing the optimisation of processes conducive to easy weight management. By making the above tools an integral and enjoyable part of our day, we will gain mastery over the area of weight management that previously may have seemed beyond our control. The knock-on positive effect on other parts of life that suffered as a result of deregulated eating is a welcome side effect.

With greater mindfulness over why we eat, we can now turn our attention to what to eat from the perspective of providing our body with optimum nutrition through a healthy, relaxed and varied diet.

Chapter Three – NUTRITION

We have purposefully not discussed nutrition yet in this book. When we formulate the desire to lose weight, diet is usually our main focus, and sometimes our only focus. We go in search of the diet plan that promises the fastest weight loss with the minimum sacrifice. However, as we have seen, restrictive practices around eating can trigger reactions that are counterproductive to the aim of losing weight and maintaining a healthy weight.

We come to diet after exploring timing and mindset in order to overturn the supreme focus on food. We come to diet having learnt that when we eat and why we eat are equally, if not more important than what we eat in our quest for easy weight management.

We have learnt that our circadian rhythm can reinforce weight management if we keep all eating within a fixed daily window during daylight hours. We have also learnt that the perfect diet cannot outsmart or outmanoeuvre subconscious psychological factors. It is important that we have uncovered what is driving our food choices and our eating habits, so that we do not set ourselves up for failure by imposing a diet that can never go head-to-head and win against physiological and psychological urges.

If your go-to diet plan involves restricting yourself for days only to find yourself emptying the fridge one evening after work, this is the alternative plan for you. Know that any previous diets that relied upon your willpower to lose weight were heavily weighted against you. You were fighting a losing battle. A list of prohibited foods

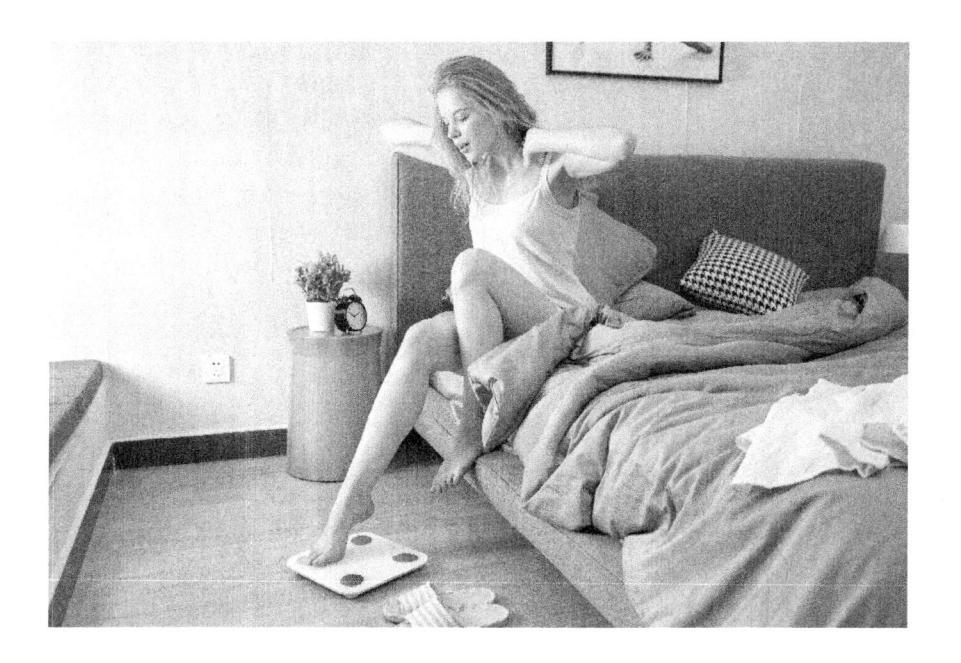

immediately sets off a mindset of deprivation and tripping up on prohibited foods can cause a landslide of abusive eating, as well as being detrimental to your self-esteem through feelings of failure. Our first step when addressing diet is to take everything off the prohibited list. No foods are banned.

Many dieting manuals before *The BODYBLISS Protocol* have simplified weight loss to a mathematical exercise of counting calories. Within the framework of the calorie-counting paradigm, weight management is reduced to balancing the equation of energy intake and energy expenditure. This very logical approach reasons that when energy consumed exceeds energy required, the body gains weight, and when energy consumed is less than energy required, the body loses weight. Energy is measured in calories. According to this theory, if one kilogram is equal to 3,500 calories, we can lose a kilogram if we can create a deficit of 3,500 calories. By creating a deficit of 500 calories a day, we can lose one kilogram of weight a week.

> How many of us have followed a strict calorie-controlled diet only to jump on the scales and find that something wasn't quite adding up and our efforts and sacrifices did not seem adequately reflected by the number on the dial?

Easy, right? Well, how many of us have tried this method and followed a strict calorie-controlled diet only to jump on the scales and find that something wasn't quite adding up and our efforts and sacrifices did not seem adequately reflected by the number on the dial? We have learnt that while we can gain a lot of weight by eating in excess of our energy requirements, we can't always lose weight just by creating an energy deficit.

Although energy intake and energy expenditure are important in weight management, the body's complexities, as well as the mind's, rarely allow us to reduce weight management to a simple mathematical equation. So, let's see what else we have to take into consideration when deciding what to eat.

Principally, *The BODYBLISS Protocol* differs from diets by its focus not on diet but instead on nutrition. Good nutrition drives satiety. Junk food often does not contain significant levels of the essential nutrients required to effectively appease hunger. In our bid to properly care for the body, we will start to choose the most nutritious food options available, the body will registers the input of protein, fat, micronutrients and fibre and trigger satiety. This is how we will work in harmony with the body's intelligence and its need for proper nutrition to reach our weight goals instead of engaging in a struggle against it.

Again, if you prefer to skip the science and jump straight into applying the principles, go to the end of this chapter to the section entitled "**NUTRITION PROTOCOL**". If you would like to understand more about why *The BODYBLISS Protocol* is so effective, read on.

Macronutrients

All food is made up of one, two or all three macronutrients: protein, carbohydrate and fat. Each macronutrient is digested differently and broken down into its constituent parts ready for absorption into the bloodstream.

Protein takes the most energy to digest (20-30% of total calories in protein eaten go towards digesting it). Next, carbohydrates lose 5-10% of their total calorie count in digestion while fats a mere 0-3%. Each macronutrient triggers the release of different hormones and signals, which have different effects on the body's tendency to use or store energy.

Diet Composition

There are a myriad of diets, which vary in terms of their proportions of macronutrients (carbohydrates, fats and protein), but generally all prescribe the creation of a daily energy deficit by caloric restriction that aims to recruit fat reserves to fill the energy gap created.

The obesity epidemic that has been swelling in recent decades correlates to increased calorie consumption. Consistently eating in excess of energy requirements will lead to excess weight. It is much easier for most people to gain weight than to lose it because of spiralling processes triggered in the body that magnify our momentum into weight gain. However, it is much more difficult to return back up the hill to healthy weight management because of the body's resistance to mobilising fat reserves.

Our social environment has fuelled this rise in obesity. Eating is not limited to mealtimes anymore. Advertising and the proliferation of all-day restaurants and coffee shops persuade us that anytime is a good time to stop and eat. So much of our social interaction at work

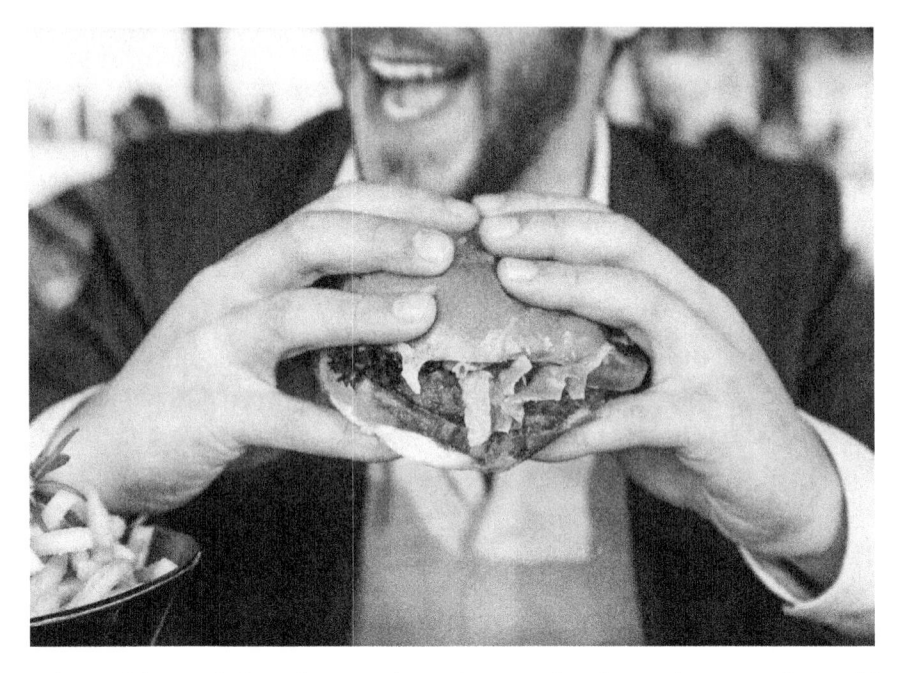

and outside work involves eating. One study showed that eating with several people increased caloric intake by up to 72%.

Highly palatable, processed foods are omnipresent and cheaper than ever before as a percentage of disposable income, whereas whole foods are relatively more expensive. This has lead to a shift in consumption from real, homemade meals produced from scratch with whole foods to ready-made, take-out, processed foods. Furthermore, the huge variety of highly palatable, junk food encourages overeating, disguising satiety through lack of real nutrition and over-stimulation of our brain's reward system.

Oversimplification of diet into calorie content has not assisted the quest for healthy weight management. The composition of the calories is equally important. Theories vary between the proportions of macronutrients required to facilitate weight management, but it is clear that micronutrient-dense foods are more desirable than the empty calories of junk food, and fats and protein are unquestionably essential components needed to provide vital compounds for the body to function correctly.

Let's analyse a few of the most common diets proposed for weight loss and management:

The Low-Fat Diet

While fat uses very little energy to be digested, it does not trigger the release of insulin. Having studied the impact of insulin in the body and the impossibility of accessing our fat reserves with high insulin levels, you may by now be thinking "so it's sugar that's making us fat, maybe more than fat itself". If you've arrived at this point, you are already ahead of the curve, and certainly ahead of most dietary guidelines published by governments in developed countries over the last few decades.

> Having studied the impact of insulin in the body and the impossibility of accessing our fat reserves with high insulin levels, you may by now be thinking "so it's sugar that's making us fat, maybe more than fat itself".

Many studies have correlated the rise of obesity with the publication of low-fat guidelines around the world, but specifically endorsed by governments in Western developed nations such as the USA and the

UK. These guidelines were prompted by a rise in heart disease, which scientists believed at the time to be related to intake of fat, especially saturated fat. The consequences of these guidelines, however, did not see a fall in heart disease and have coincided instead with an obesity epidemic in the countries where these guidelines were most actively promoted.

The low-fat diet adopted often favoured processed foods that were lower in fat than their full-fat counterparts, but higher in sugar. It is estimated that sugar consumption in the USA increased by approximately 30% between 1980 and 2000, while the incidence of obesity almost tripled. Natural fats, such as lard and butter, were replaced with hydrogenated fats like margarine and vegetable oils. It was later proven that these trans fats increase bad (LDL) cholesterol levels and lower good (HDL) cholesterol levels, thus increasing the risk of developing heart disease and stroke. They are also associated with a higher risk of developing type 2 diabetes.

Other fats, in particular omega-3 fatty acids (found in fatty fish, walnuts and flaxseed oil), have since been found to be important in preventing and managing heart disease. They also have the ability to increase levels of leptin, which diminishes appetite and food intake. Omega-3 fatty acids can also improve insulin resistance, inflammation and heart disease risk factors.

> The aim is to return to a youthful metabolic efficiency in which the body alternates between glucose and fat as its principal fuel. It can only achieve this if its glucose supply is regularly depleted on a daily basis.

Studies have shown that fat oxidation is higher in prepubescent children than in adults. This may suggest that either children have higher fat requirements than adults, perhaps because of typically higher energy expenditure that exhausts glucose faster than in adults, or that their metabolism switches more efficiently between the two.

Puberty signals a reduction in fat oxidation and insulin sensitivity. The aim is to return to the youthful metabolic efficiency in which the body alternates between glucose and fat as its principal fuel. It can only achieve this if its glucose supply is regularly depleted on a daily basis. So, let's investigate low-sugar, high-fat diets instead.

The High-Fat Diet
The so-called French paradox has puzzled scientists for many years. How could the French eat butter, cream and full-fat cheese and still remain slim with lower rates of heart disease, while the American population was dramatically reducing fat intake and yet were getting fatter and fatter and suffering from higher rates of heart disease?

In recent years, studies have shown that there are significant health benefits to be gleaned from increasing fat intake, while simultaneously reducing carbohydrate intake. These benefits include:

> There are significant health benefits to be gleaned from increasing fat intake, while simultaneously reducing carbohydrate intake.

- Increased satiety by elevating leptin levels and reducing ghrelin;
- Better insulin sensitivity and improvements in type 2 diabetes;
- Increases in good cholesterol levels – saturated fat does not raise saturated fat levels in the blood, excess carbohydrates are more likely to do so;
- Reduced total food intake, improved metabolism and easier weight loss;
- Improved cognitive function and mood;
- Reduced inflammation, especially with increased intake of omega-3 fatty acids;
- Improved blood vessel health and lower risk of cardiovascular disease.

The above benefits are in stark contrast to common understanding about fat. Many of the dangers associated with fat, and in particular saturated fat, are actually more accurately associated with higher intakes of sugar and refined carbohydrates, which increase lipogenesis, triglyceride levels in the blood and LDL cholesterol levels.

Like protein, fat is not an optional, but an essential component of a healthy diet. Fat-soluble vitamins, such as vitamins A, D and E, need the presence of fat in order to be absorbed from the food we eat. Fat is also needed to build strong, healthy cell membranes, the walls of each cell, and the sheaths surrounding nerves. It is essential for blood clotting, muscle movement, healthy skin, immune function and hormone synthesis.

Recently, many studies have applauded the benefits of a very high fat diet that has come to be known as the ketogenic diet. The ketogenic diet was originally used as a therapy for epilepsy in the 1920s and is today being studied as a possible therapy for various conditions, including diabetes, polycystic ovary syndrome, neurological diseases, cancer and cardiovascular disease.

> The ketogenic diet was originally used as a therapy for epilepsy in the 1920s and is today being studied as a possible therapy for various conditions, including diabetes, polycystic ovary syndrome, neurological diseases, cancer and cardiovascular disease.

Ketogenic diets are characterised by a very low daily intake of carbohydrates (usually less than 50g a day) and high levels of fat. After a day or so on the ketogenic diet, glucose levels are exhausted. The body then turns to fat reserves for energy production. Ketone bodies (acetoacetate, b-hydroxybutyric acid and acetone, produced from the breakdown of fatty acids) provide an alternative energy source. Unlike free fatty acids, ketone bodies are able to cross the blood-brain barrier and provide a fuel source for the central nervous system, which usually depends upon glucose. Blood glucose levels are kept within normal levels by glucose formed from glucogenic amino acids and from the glycerol backbone of triglycerides through gluconeogenesis.

As touched upon above, ketogenic diets appear to improve blood lipid profiles and consequently reduce cardiovascular disease risk factors. Not only is the level of triglycerides reduced, but there is also a marked reduction in total cholesterol levels. The ketogenic diet appears to increase levels of high-density lipoprotein (HDL) cholesterol and increases the size and volume of low-density lipoprotein (LDL) cholesterol particles reducing their atherogenicity and the risk of cardiovascular disease. As insulin is required to activate a key enzyme in cholesterol biosynthesis (3-hydroxy-3-methylglutaryl–CoA), a high-glucose diet that triggers high levels of insulin favours increased endogenous cholesterol synthesis.

Weight loss on ketogenic diets has been ascribed to the satiating effect of higher fat and protein intake, a reduction in lipogenesis and an increase in lipolysis, from reduced insulin levels. Due to the reduction in glucose intake and insulin secretion on a ketogenic diet, improvements have also been shown in cases of insulin resistance, type 2 diabetes and obesity.

The Low-Sugar Diet
As we have seen, cellular energy metabolism depends upon two main energy substrates: glucose and fatty acids. The proportions of this fuel mix are determined by glucose availability and insulin secretion. When both are high, glucose is used preferentially to generate energy and lipogenesis is stimulated, increasing body fat. Fatty acids are used for energy production when energy expenditure is increased, during long bouts of exercise for example, and when glucose availability is reduced.

> Proponents of low carbohydrate diets argue that it is impossible to reduce fat reserves in the presence of insulin.

Proponents of low carbohydrate diets argue that it is impossible to reduce fat reserves in the presence of insulin. Insulin's function is to regulate blood sugar levels. While there is excess glucose in the blood, insulin is present to aid its transport into cells, where it can be transformed into energy. Even in the face of insulin resistance, fat cells remain receptive to insulin, allowing it to clear excess sugar from the blood, by pouring it into fat cells for storage, before it can create problems.

Therefore, while the release of insulin is continually triggered by carbohydrate-rich meals and snacks, the body is busy dealing with the blood glucose situation and does not even get a chance to access its fat reserves. Any excess intake will also be immediately stored as extra fat. In order to start using fat reserves for energy production, there needs to be a drop in insulin. In the absence of insulin, glucagon activates lipolysis and fat reserves can be accessed, drawn upon and reduced.

The anabolic effects of insulin have led many to become proponents of a low-carbohydrate diet. The theory revolves around the weight-loss potential of keeping insulin secretion to a minimum. Proponents of this theory negate the calories in/calories out model and propose that fat loss is achieved only by reducing carbohydrate intake to such an extent that insulin is minimized and the body is forced to use fat from the diet or from reserves to fuel metabolic needs.

These diets range from the renowned Atkins diet, which is high in both fat and protein and seeks to abolish carbohydrate intake, to the ketogenic diets, which are high in fat, low in protein and very low in carbohydrates.

The key, as is often the case, is a balanced approach, which taps the best of both worlds. While simply depending upon caloric restriction is difficult (especially in the face of countering processes, such as reductions in BMR and increases in hunger cues), excess intake from fat and protein will still convert into weight gain. Any diet that cuts out a whole food group, whether it is low-carbohydrate or low-fat, can translate into an energy deficit that promotes weight loss, but may not be ideal for health.

> Fat loss is achieved only by reducing carbohydrate intake to such an extent that insulin is minimized and the body is forced to use fat from the diet or from reserves to fuel metabolic needs.

However, rather than tracking calories and macronutrients and the effects of what we eat on insulin secretion, which limits our focus on nutrition, it is more important to track instead how many times we stimulate insulin secretion in a day and start with our Chapter One focus on timing. As we saw in Chapter One, insulin clearing is key to fat loss. Low carbohydrate diets are one method to achieve insulin clearing, but insulin clearing is also achieved by leaving sufficient time in between meals.

The High-Sugar Diet
Our sugar consumption has skyrocketed in recent decades; we snack more, drink more sugary beverages and grab convenience food on the go, which is usually packed with sugar. As previously mentioned, the low-fat focus facilitated the substitution of sugar for fat in many cases and, contrary to fat, sugar is not as efficient at promoting satiety. Some recent studies have linked fructose consumption, which increased by 26% between 1970 and 1997, to the rise in type 2 diabetes and obesity.

Consumption of sodas and soft drinks that are high in fructose has increased significantly in the past few decades. Just 2 cans of soft drinks can supply 50g of fructose and 200 calories, more than 10% of the daily energy requirements for an average woman. Many breakfast cereals, baked goods, condiments and prepared desserts are sweetened with high-fructose corn syrup. Fructose consumed alone does not stimulate insulin secretion and, as leptin levels are regulated by insulin, leptin levels are not increased either. This results in a combined anti-satiety effect. Fructose is also an unregulated source of both glycerol-3-phosphate and acetyl-CoA for hepatic lipogenesis.

> Studies have shown that a single daily serving of a sugar-sweetened beverage is linked to a more than 60% increased risk of obesity in children.

Studies have shown that a single daily serving of a sugar-sweetened beverage is linked to a more than 60% increased risk of obesity in children. High fructose intake is also linked to insulin resistance and hyperlipidaemia.

A high-carbohydrate diet, rich in glucose rather than fructose has different effects. Insulin and leptin levels increase following glucose consumption and ghrelin levels fall, so there is a satiety effect that is absent with fructose consumption. All high-sugar diets trigger high levels of insulin release. If the diet produces high spikes of insulin regularly then, as we have seen, this is a recipe for insulin resistance, type 2 diabetes, weight gain and obesity.

Fructose from fruit and vegetables does not have the same deleterious effect on insulin sensitivity, glucose tolerance and hyperlipidaemia as sucrose or high-fructose corn syrup because the levels of fructose are lower and clothed in high levels of fibre, micronutrients and antioxidants.

The High-Fibre Diet
Whole foods that are rich in fibre, such as fruit, vegetables, nuts, whole grains and legumes, increase satiety and regulate blood sugar levels by slowing down the absorption of glucose into the blood

stream. It is the blood sugar spikes caused by refined sugar that stress our insulinic response and escalate weight management issues, such as insulin resistance, type 2 diabetes and obesity. Fibre stretches the stomach, slows its emptying rate and activates satiety hormones.

Fibre is also essential for optimum gastrointestinal health. It prevents constipation, it ferments in the bowel to produce short-chain fatty acids (the anti-inflammatory and anti-carcinogenic primary energy source for colonic cells), sustaining the microbiome and increasing feelings of fullness.

High-fibre foods also tend to be more nutritious, especially when compared to the highly palatable processed foods we crave that are high in calories, fat, sugar and salt, and very low in fibre, such as cakes, pastries, biscuits, pizza, crisps, soda, ice cream, chocolate, white bread, pasta and rice. These foods are less efficient at curbing satiety and create addictive circuits in our brain's reward system pathways.

The High-Protein Diet

We know that protein is an essential macronutrient that provides the body with the amino acids it requires for the structure, function and regulation of its tissues and organs. Recommendations on daily intake vary according to level of physical activity, but are around 0.8g per kilogram of weight. So, if you weigh 60kg, you'll need around 48g of protein a day. An insufficient supply of protein in the diet causes a loss of muscle mass, a weakened immune system, compromised organ

> An insufficient supply of protein in the diet causes a loss of muscle mass, a weakened immune system, compromised organ function and ultimately death. A low-protein diet is, therefore, not recommended. Sufficient protein intake is vital for optimum health.

function and ultimately death. A low-protein diet is, therefore, not recommended. Sufficient protein intake is vital for optimum health.

A protein-rich diet guards against muscle loss, which is highly probable during a calorie-restricted diet or intensive training programme. Eating a protein-rich meal promotes satiety more than fat and carbohydrates, reduces food intake at the following meal and is, therefore, an essential component of effective weight management.

Some diets, such as the Atkins diet, permit high levels of protein, but ban nutrient-rich foods such as fruit and some vegetables. Some studies suggest that high-protein diets cause possible kidney damage due to high levels of nitrogen excretion during protein metabolism, which can cause an increase in glomerular pressure and hyperfiltration. However, there is not a proven link except where renal damage already exists. The healthiest choice, however, lies not in these extreme regimes, but in a more balanced approach.

An Optimum Diet

The research is very divided between the efficacy of each of the above-mentioned diets at promoting healthy weight maintenance and reducing all-cause mortality. Some studies show that low carbohydrate diets increase mortality, while others show that they reduce mortality and there is no consistent superiority proven in terms of weight loss. What is evident is that the body is adaptive metabolically to different proportions of macronutrients.

Therefore, rather than disproportionately favouring one macronutrient over another, it would seem that a more balanced approach is the healthiest route. The Mediterranean diet has consistently been shown to outclass other diet programmes in terms of weight management, cardiovascular health, all-cause mortality and cognitive health. The Mediterranean diet as the name suggests is a diet common to Mediterranean countries that is high in nutrient-rich fresh fruits and vegetables, contains moderate amounts of meat and dairy products, very few processed foods and some red wine and coffee. It is also rich in olive oil and omega-3 fatty acids from fish.

Coffee has been shown in some studies to increase the release of the satiety hormone PYY, with effects lasting up to three hours. Coffee has also been shown to improve insulin sensitivity. In Mediterranean countries, consumption of coffee is traditionally higher than consumption of sweetened beverages and sodas. Hydration is also key, but with water rather than other beverages. Indeed, a study showed that drinking two glasses of water prior to a meal reduced food intake by 22% as the gastric distension triggers satiety signals in the brain.

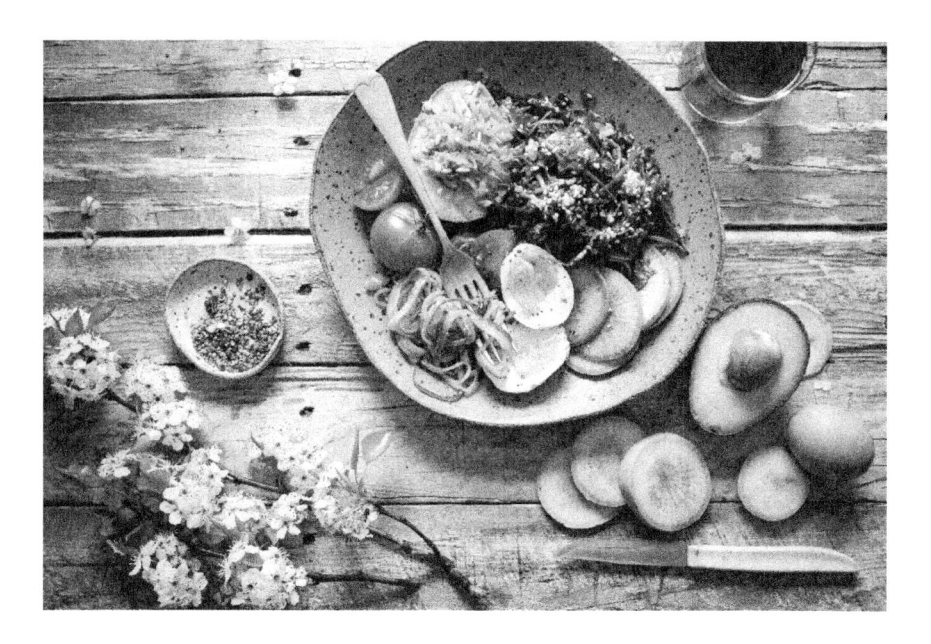

Studies have found that many of the negative effects of excess dietary fat can be neutralized by a significant intake of omega-3 fatty acids. In particular, elevated levels of free fatty acids and triglycerides in the blood accelerate insulin resistance, but are inversely correlated with omega-3 intake. High triglyceride levels may be driven by excess fat intake, but also by excess intake of simple carbohydrates, sucrose and fructose especially, which are converted into triglycerides by the liver.

Healthy dietary choices and diet composition facilitate easy weight management while poor choices can shunt weight management off course. Below we have a table that collates the information regarding certain factors that will reinforce appetite signals conducive to efficient weight management:

	Effects
Protein	<ul><li>Inhibits NPY</li><li>Inhibits ghrelin</li><li>Inhibits insulin</li><li>Stimulates CCK</li><li>Stimulates PYY</li><li>Stimulates GLP-1</li></ul>
Low carbohydrate intake	<ul><li>Inhibits ghrelin</li><li>Inhibits insulin</li><li>Stimulates PYY</li></ul>
Fat	<ul><li>Inhibits insulin</li><li>Stimulates CCK</li></ul>
Prebiotics	<ul><li>Inhibit NPY</li><li>Stimulate CCK</li><li>Stimulate PYY</li><li>Stimulate GLP-1</li></ul>
Vitamin D	<ul><li>Inhibits ghrelin</li></ul>
Coffee	<ul><li>Stimulates PYY</li></ul>
Magnesium and Chromium	<ul><li>Improve insulin sensitivity</li></ul>

Anti-inflammatories, curcumin	e.g.	• Stimulate GLP-1 • Stimulate leptin
Catechins		• Inhibit insulin • Stimulate GLP-1 • Stimulate leptin
Oestrogen		• Inhibits MCH • Stimulates leptin • Stimulates insulin
Sleep		• Stimulates leptin
Exercise		• Inhibits insulin • Stimulates leptin

Fig. 1: Balancing factors for optimum weight management

Protein has been shown to be very effective at satisfying hunger by increasing the secretion of satiety hormones and increasing leptin sensitivity. It also increases the thermic effect of food digestion, improves glucose homeostasis and prevents the loss of muscle mass common during dieting. Specific amino acids, such as l-arginine and l-lysine, have also been shown to cause satiating effects in isolation by increasing plasma levels of GLP-1 and PYY.

Another method of reversing insulin resistance is the insulin clearing method outlined previously. The key is to cut down the number of times per day that insulin is triggered. If someone is used to constantly snacking, this will have to be done gradually in order to avoid conditions such as hypoglycaemia in which insulin is overexpressed and drives blood glucose levels too low.

There have been some positive results in sensitising insulin receptors in the body through the ingestion of herbal products. The most successful of these have been berberine, turmeric, ginger, apple cider vinegar, green tea, resveratrol and garlic. The amino acid l-carnitine, as well as acetyl-l-carnitine, have also shown promising insulin-sensitising properties.

As highlighted previously, insulin resistance is a driver for chronic inflammation in the body, which exacerbates leptin resistance and inhibits satiety signals, such as GLP-1. Curcumin and catechins are useful against this factor, as is consumption of omega-3 fatty acids.

Both soluble and non-soluble fibre in the diet is beneficial for gastrointestinal health. Fibre slows down the rate of glucose absorption and increases satiety through the perception of fullness and through the stimulation of satiety hormones, such as PYY and GLP-1. The short chain fatty acids generated by the intestinal microbiota from indigestible fibre directly stimulate PYY.

Micronutrients
While the body is adaptive to different proportions of macronutrients in the diet, it must receive adequate amounts of fat and protein. Equally, micronutrients are not optional but fundamentally essential for health and the optimum functioning of the body, including effective weight management. Certain micronutrients have a greater role than others in the processes essential to healthy weight management. We will run through some that have been studied for their positive impact on weight loss and weight management.

- Chromium enhances the action of insulin, thus helping the body to maintain normal blood glucose levels.
- Choline is essential for normal metabolism, lipid transportation, methylation reactions and neurotransmitter synthesis.

- Serum vitamin D levels are inversely related to BMI and body fat mass. Vitamin D is claimed to inhibit lipogenesis and fat storage. It regulates serotonin synthesis and increases testosterone levels, both of which aid weight management.
- Iodine is critical for healthy thyroid function, metabolism and thermogenesis. It also helps reverse insulin resistance.
- Niacin (vitamin B3) reduces LDL cholesterol, triglyceride and lipoprotein levels, while increasing HDL cholesterol levels. It plays a vital role in cellular metabolism, mitochondrial function and DNA repair.
- Magnesium is essential to the generation and transportation of energy. It is useful in cases of fatigue, improving exercise performance and counteracting insomnia. It activates enzymes essential for protein and carbohydrate metabolism and it is required for the synthesis and function of DNA. It also helps counteract insulin resistance.
- Copper is an endogenous regulator of lipolysis. Low levels of copper may reduce thyroid function and BMR, as well as increase cholesterol levels, fatigue and reduce nerve conductivity.
- Coenzyme Q10 plays an important role in the generation of energy in mitochondria. Endogenous levels have been seen to diminish with age. It improves exercise performance, insulin resistance, antioxidant protection; it regulates blood glucose levels and has cardioprotective properties.
- L-carnitine, or acetyl-l-carnitine, is crucial for the transportation of fatty acids into the mitochondria and efficient energy production. By inducing fatty acid oxidation, carnitine can be a useful aid to weight loss. It also supports mitochondrial health, protecting the mitochondria from age-related deterioration, and it has a positive effect on cognitive function. Some studies have shown positive effects of carnitine supplementation on exercise performance, in particular on resistance and recovery, as well as improving insulin sensitivity.

- Curcumin is well known for its anti-inflammatory properties. Some studies have highlighted the key role of inflammation in obesity as both a driver and a result. Inflammation interferes with hypothalamic signalling. Curcumin boosts brain function, serotonin and dopamine levels, endogenous antioxidant action and also has cardioprotective properties.
- Some studies suggest that the high-fibre Irvingia Gabonensis seed reduces blood glucose levels, total cholesterol and triglycerides while increasing HDL cholesterol. It is thus purported to improve insulin resistance, type 2 diabetes and facilitate weight management.
- Green tea contains caffeine, which activates some lipolysis and is purported to improve exercise performance. However, it is green tea's high catechin content that distinguishes it, in particular epigallocatechin gallate (EPCG), which boosts antioxidant action and metabolism, as well as improving insulin sensitivity and glucose tolerance.
- Resveratrol, a phytochemical found in grapes and berries, has antioxidant, neuroprotective, cardioprotective, hepatoprotective and anti-inflammatory properties. It improves insulin sensitivity, cholesterol levels and metabolism.
- Sulforaphane, found in broccoli and other cruciferous vegetables, is an antioxidant and an anti-inflammatory (it actively inhibits NF-kB and suppresses TNF-α-induced inflammation). It encourages lipolysis, normalises blood glucose levels and improves insulin sensitivity. Some studies have noted a synergistic effect with curcumin.
- Fibre induces satiety, improves insulin sensitivity, cholesterol levels, metabolic health and gut health.

Do We Need Supplements?
Ideally, we would integrate all the nutrients the body needs from a healthy, balanced diet rich in fresh fruits, vegetables, whole grains and healthy protein. Indeed, nature's bounty is a far superior method for our bodies to receive nutrition than in pill form. Why would we

not prefer to eat a bowl of blueberries than take a pill containing blueberry extract, for example? Not only is it more pleasurable to eat blueberries in their natural state, but also the nutritional value, in terms of live phytochemicals, such as pterostilbene (similar to resveratrol) and flavonoids, the rich mix of vitamins and minerals and the healthy fibre, can never be fully replicated in a pill. Why, then, are we consuming more supplements than ever?

Many of us turn to food supplements as a back-up plan to compensate for possible shortfalls in our diets. Our lifestyles may be such that we cannot guarantee healthy dietary choices every day. However, even if our diets are healthy and balanced, do we still need supplements? Are there still reasons, circumstances and conditions in which we may not be getting all the nutrients we need from our diets?

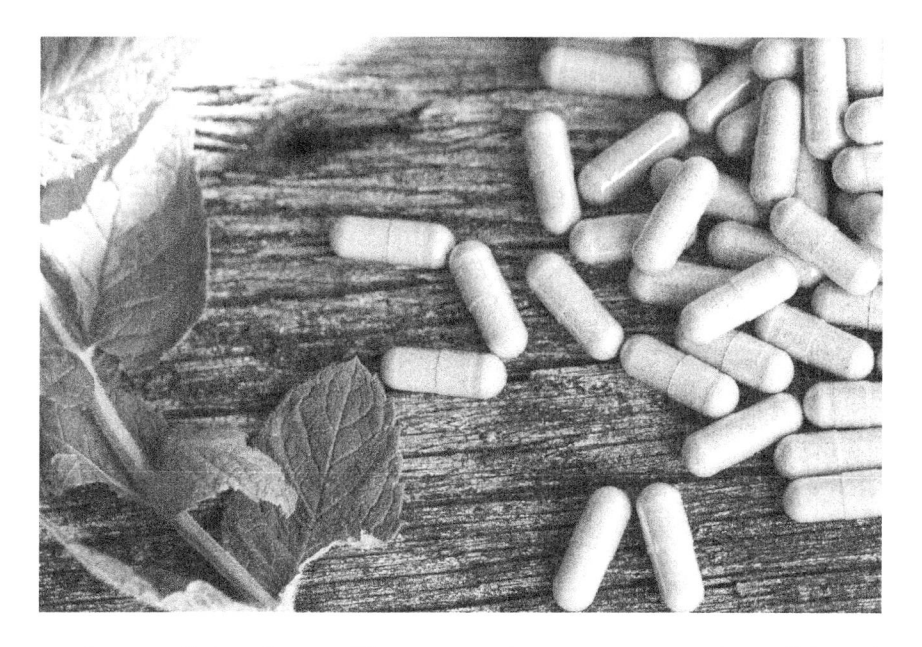

The answer unfortunately is yes and overwhelming research extols their use and benefits. Crops grown decades ago were much richer in vitamins and minerals than they are today. Ever more intensive agricultural methods are stripping our soils of vital nutrients. A study tracking the nutrient decline in 20 crops between 1930 and 1980, found that the average calcium content had declined by 19%, iron by 22% and potassium by 14%.

Fruit and vegetables are often picked before they have ripened and reached their full nutrient potential in order to be shipped many miles away. Foods are often refined, processed and packaged in such a way that depletes their original levels of nutrients further.

For all these reasons, the food we eat is not as rich in nutrients as it used to be and we would need a much greater quantity to get the same nutritional value as we would have integrated from less decades ago.

Levels of stress, poor gut health and alcohol consumption are three more factors that may deplete our nutrient levels further, which all reinforces the advantages of integrating our diets with extra nutrients from supplements. We will explore which supplements may be of highest value for optimum health and easy weight management in our "**NUTRITION PROTOCOL**" later in this chapter.

Be conscious of the glycaemic load
The glycaemic load of food is an estimate of how much the food will raise our blood glucose levels after eating it. Foods with a high glycaemic count are those (usually refined carbohydrates such as white bread, pasta and sweets) that are rapidly digested into sugar and pour into the bloodstream triggering a rapid rise in blood glucose levels and consequently a rapid spike in insulin.

Fibre slows down the transport of sugar into the bloodstream, so complex carbohydrates, such as brown rice and whole wheat bread, are digested at a slower rate than their white, refined counterparts, so insulin is triggered less forcefully. If a meal contains protein and fat together with the carbohydrates, digestion is slowed down further and the rate at which sugar enters the bloodstream is slower and the insulin response is more balanced.

Therefore, we need to be conscious of the glycaemic value of the food we eat so as not to spike insulin release excessively. We can slow down a sugar rush, by balancing a meal in terms of protein and fat content. It is difficult to overeat protein or fat, but it is easy to overeat carbohydrates, as they do not have the same effect on satiety signals in the body. Protein and fat are essential, carbohydrate is not, but some carbohydrates, in particular vegetables and fruit, integrate many healthy nutrients.

> If a meal contains protein and fat together with carbohydrates, digestion is slowed down and the rate at which sugar enters the bloodstream is slower and the insulin response is more balanced.

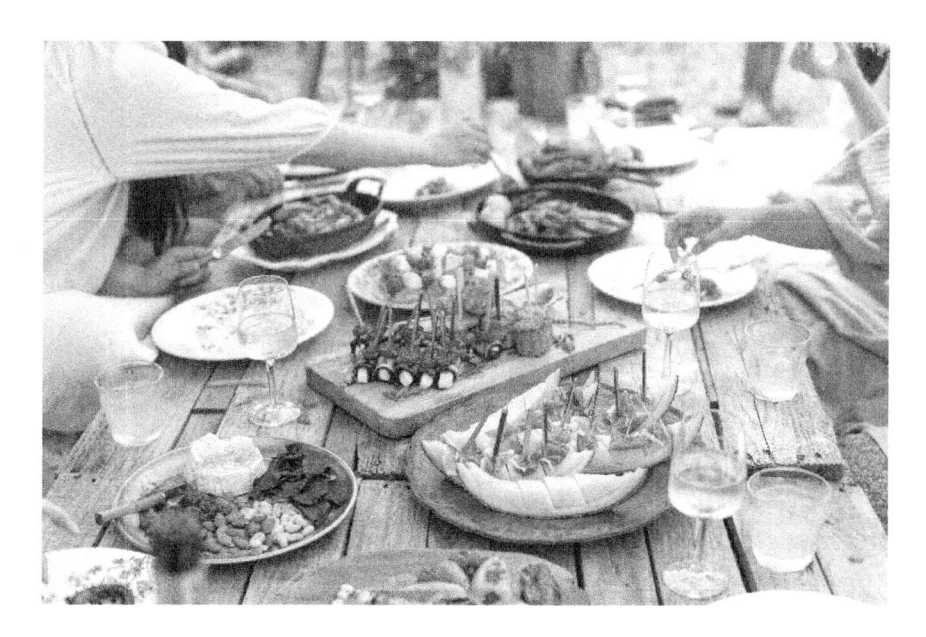

If we want to indulge in sweets and desserts, the timing of their consumption is important. Eaten after a meal, their effect on blood glucose levels will be slowed down compared to eating them as a snack between meals.

Understanding Nutrition
So, we have learnt that contrary to popular belief, a calorie is not just a calorie, its composition (macro- and micronutrient content) is key in terms of the metabolic effect it will have on the body, as is the timing of its consumption. In terms of insulin secretion alone, sugar and simple carbohydrates will trigger a high insulinic response. Protein, complex carbohydrates, fruit and vegetables have a lower insulinic response and fat alone does not produce an insulinic response at all. Insulin is important for delivering nutrients into cells, but too much can create problems. Therefore, the composition of our diet should mirror this need for balance.

Constantly triggering insulin with highly palatable, fatty and sugary snacks is a fast track to insulin resistance, type 2 diabetes and obesity. A better approach favours nutritious food over empty, junk food calories. Fruit, vegetables, omega-3 fatty acids, high-quality protein sources, whole grains and fats are all essential components of a healthy diet. The fibre, fat and protein induce satiety, which is crucial for sustaining a weight loss programme. If we desire to eat junk food or sugary treats, it is best to mix them in a meal with healthier, high-fibre or protein-rich foods that will blunt the insulin spike usually triggered by such foods.

> Caloric restriction reduces BMR because it is interpreted by the body as a sign of scarcity in the environment and pushes the body into energy-saving mode.

Caloric restriction reduces BMR because it is interpreted by the body as a sign of scarcity in the environment and pushes the body into energy-saving mode. A lower BMR means that the body can survive on less food. Therefore, consuming less food will not create the energy deficit required to lose weight, it will instead trigger within the body an adaptive response to the reduction of input, which further reduces its requirements for energy. In order to lose weight, the caloric input must be reduced further and further, triggering further falls in BMR. This is a losing battle. However, caloric restriction has been the main diet recommendation for weight loss to date. A caloric deficit seems to be an obvious essential prerequisite for weight loss and, in broad terms, it is, but it is also important to maintain BMR as, if we don't, caloric restriction will drive down BMR and it will become harder and harder to lose weight or indeed to maintain a healthy level of nutrition without putting weight on.

While insulin is still being triggered and in our system, despite caloric restriction and even with small snacks, we are not able to successfully access the fat reserves that could fill the energy deficit while maintaining BMR because insulin inhibits lipolysis. When we stop snacking, insulin and blood glucose levels will finally drop sufficiently to stimulate glucagon release, which will mobilise fat reserves. The balanced dance between glucagon and insulin is vital for healthy weight management and, therefore, the balance between eating and not eating is a key tool.

Good nutrition is vital for easy weight management because it drives satiety and it ensures optimum health by fulfilling all the body's nutritional requirements. As we learnt in Chapter One, timing is essential in ensuring that we can eat a healthy, nutritious and sufficient diet without running into weight issues. By maintaining a feeding window of under 12 hours, BMR is sustained, dietary failings are mitigated and weight management and optimum health are achieved. No foods are off the menu, but with feeding restricted to a time window of under 12 hours and all

> Good nutrition is vital for easy weight management because it drives satiety and it ensures optimum health by fulfilling all the body's nutritional requirements.

physiological and psychological urges balanced, we will generally tend towards healthier choices for our diet.

The "**NUTRITION PROTOCOL**" proposed is easily compatible with any lifestyle. It does not involve calorie-counting or constant deliberations over what is permitted or not because good timing and a balanced mindset have removed the diabolic influence of any particular foods.

NUTRITION PROTOCOL

By practising time-restricted feeding (TRF), we have learnt that the deleterious effects of dietary failings within the 8-to-12-hour feeding window are mitigated. However, having also learnt how to balance the physiological and psychological aspects of appetite, we are now more inclined to make the healthiest, most nutritious dietary choices to best care for the body. The following steps will remove the usual misery that comes with going on a diet and make attaining and maintaining ideal weight easy and enjoyable.

Step One: Balance and Rhythm

Optimum health and easy weight management were never achieved through extremes and unsustainable diet regimes; they are achieved through balance and respecting the body's natural rhythms and cycles. If you have been practising TRF, you should be regularly clearing insulin levels and activating a shift from glucose metabolism to fat metabolism, that is, from fuelling your body with sugar to regularly mobilising your fat reserves. So, the following are added tips for even better balance and rhythm and, consequently, optimum health and weight management:
- ✓ Drink 1-2 glasses of water before a meal;
- ✓ Eat no more than 2 or 3 meals a day;
- ✓ Make lunch the biggest meal of the day;
- ✓ Balance the macronutrient content of your meals to always include protein and fat.

Step Two: Supplements
In order to ensure that we have all our nutritional requirements covered, as well as some specific nutrients to optimise easy weight management, the following supplements are recommended:
- ✓ A high-quality, broad spectrum multi-vitamin supplement, like MAGNESSENCE® from FIREBIRD®, which, as well as covering all of our vitamin and mineral requirements, also contains many healthy botanicals, such as turmeric, resveratrol and chlorella;
- ✓ A high-quality weight loss supplement, such as BODYBLISS® from FIREBIRD®, which contains nutrients that specifically support weight management, including green tea, chromium, magnesium, niacin, acetyl-l-carnitine, kelp, irvingia gabonensis, 5-HTP, tyrosine, coenzyme Q10, l-citrulline, ginseng, apple cider vinegar, turmeric, cayenne, grape seed and green coffee extract.

Step Three: Cook from scratch
We all need to find a number of healthy, go-to meals that work according to our individual taste and interest in cooking. The term healthy is used to indicate natural produce that provides the body with excellent nourishment and nutrition. The following recipes are intended solely as indications of what could be considered healthy food and possibly to provide inspiration to create your own easy and quick meals. Easy and quick is essential to avoid falling back on ready-made, heavily processed and chemical-laden options. Also, when choosing what to eat, make sure that you always integrate a good source of protein.

Many of the recipes, as well as being healthy, are also happy, that is, they contain nutrients that upgrade our serotonin levels:
- B vitamins (brown rice, poultry, eggs, green leafy vegetables, nuts and seeds, tuna, salmon, shrimp, peas, legumes, meat and corn);
- Calcium (dairy products, sardines, salmon, green leafy vegetables, sesame seeds and almonds);

- Magnesium (green leafy vegetables, salmon, sesame seeds, brown rice, avocado, apples, almonds and chocolate);
- Tryptophan (cottage cheese, peanuts, tuna, almonds, shellfish, salmon, poultry, eggs, milk and seeds).

Breakfast/Snack Options

The recipe section contains some sweet and savoury options depending upon what you like for breakfast or if you delay breakfast, these options can work equally well as a brunch or as a light supper.

- Apples with peanut butter or cheese
- Poached eggs on avocado toast
- Cottage cheese with flaxseed oil and honey
- Greek yoghurt with fruit (banana, mango, berries, etc.)
- Porridge with nuts and seeds
- Granola
- Flapjacks
- Chia pudding
- Banana muffins

Lunch/Dinner Options

- Soup (choose from the options that follow or invent your own version)
- Omelette with salad or green beans
- Salad or vegetables with protein, for example, Sardines with cherry tomatoes and roast vegetables, Salade Niçoise, Caprese salad, Salmon with asparagus, Tagliata with salad and/or roast vegetables, Chicken Goujons with salad and/or vegetables
- Thai curry with rice
- Pasta with protein, for example, Tagliatelle al Salmone
- Dips, such as guacamole or hummus, with crudités
- Dessert options include chocolate torte, chocolate mousse and ice lollies.

Flapjacks
200ml Coconut oil
500g Porridge Oats
200g Dried Fruit (coconut, nuts, seeds, sultanas, cranberries)
12 tablespoons of Maple Syrup

1. Line a baking tray and preheat the oven to 150C
2. Melt the coconut oil and mix with all the other ingredients in a bowl
3. Pour the mixture out onto the tray and press flat
4. Bake for 20-25 minutes until golden brown
5. Cool in the tin before cutting into squares

Granola
150ml Coconut oil
500g Porridge Oats
200g Dried Fruit (coconut, nuts, seeds, sultanas, cranberries)
12 tablespoons of Maple Syrup

1. Prepare as with flapjacks above, but spread out on the baking tray instead of pressing flat
2. Bake in the oven for 25-30 minutes, stirring regularly until golden brown
3. Cool completely before storing

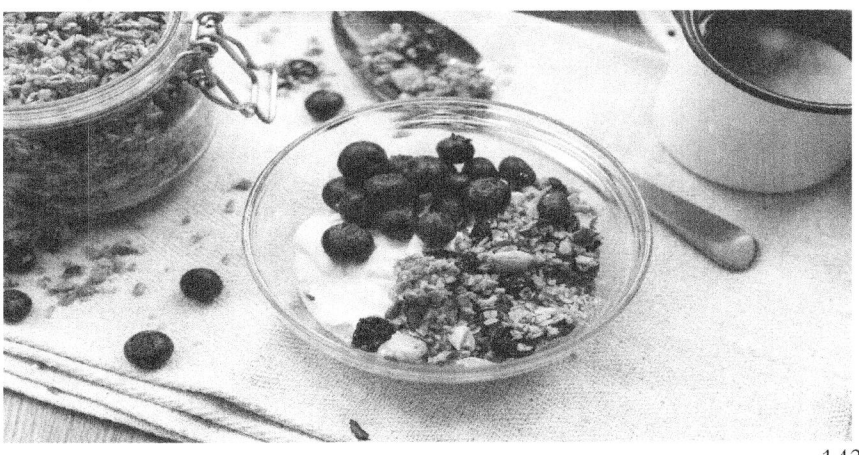

Chia Pudding

1½ cups milk (any – cows, goats, coconut, almond or cashew)
½ cup chia seeds
Sweetener of choice (stevia, maple syrup, honey)
Fruit and nuts of choice

1. Add the milk, chia seeds and sweetener to a bowl and mix together well so that there are no lumps;
2. Cover and refrigerate overnight (or for at least 6 hours) until the chia pudding develops a thick and creamy consistency;
3. Enjoy as is, or layer with fresh fruit and/or nuts.

Greek Yoghurt

Greek yoghurt can replace the chia pudding for a similar breakfast or snack.
Choose plain, natural Greek yoghurt and sweeten with stevia, maple syrup or honey and add fruit, nuts and seeds.

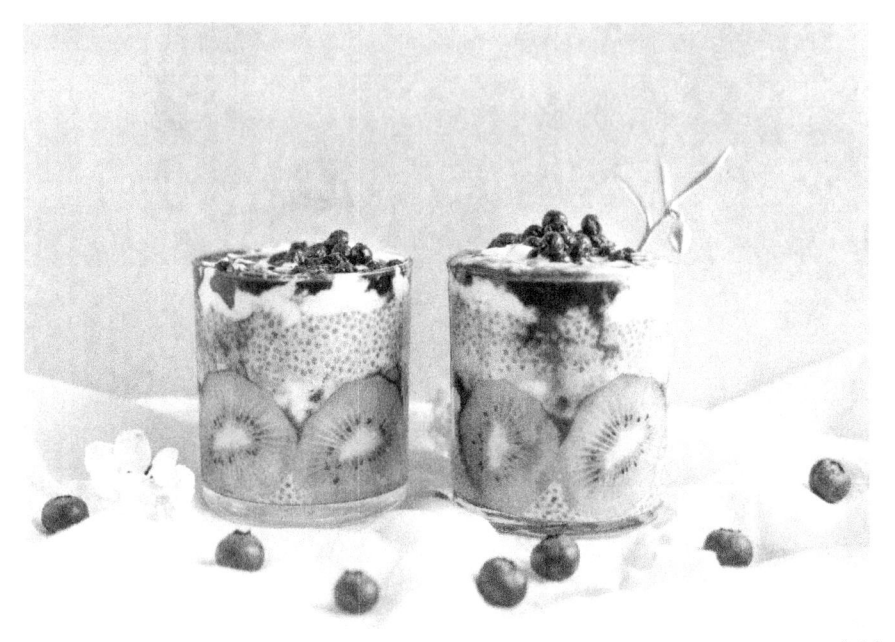

Banana Muffins

⅓ cup melted coconut oil or extra-virgin olive oil
½ cup maple syrup or honey
2 eggs or 60ml chickpea water
3 mashed ripe bananas
¼ cup milk of choice or water
1 teaspoon of baking soda
½ teaspoon cinnamon
1½ cup of rice or oat flour
1 cup of ground almonds
½ cup of Greek yoghurt
Extras: chopped nuts, berries, cocao nibs

1. Preheat oven to 180C
2. Line muffin tray with paper cases
3. In a large bowl, mix together all the wet ingredients
4. Fold in the powdered ingredients and any extras.
5. Divide the batter between the muffin cups.
6. Bake for 20-25 minutes until a skewer inserted comes out clean.
7. Cool muffins on a cooling rack before eating.

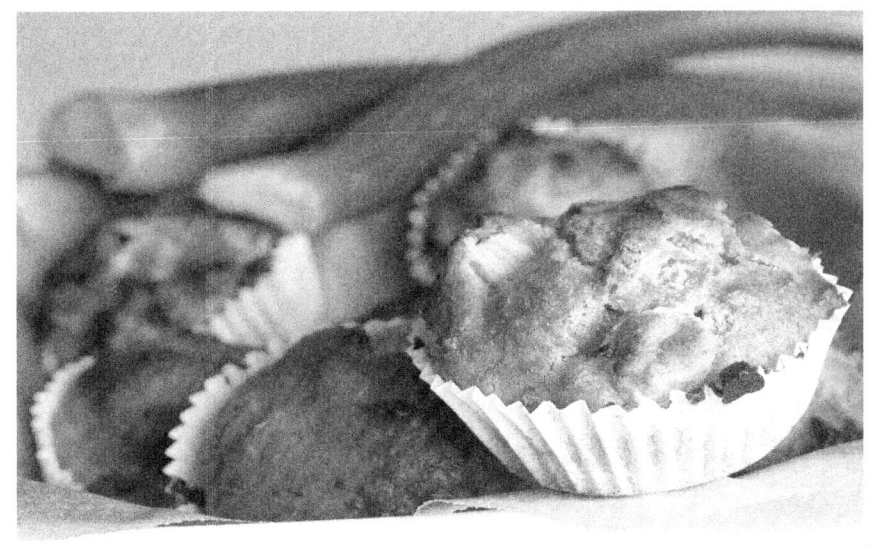

Salade Niçoise

Lettuce
Tomatoes
Spring onions
Green beans
Hard-boiled eggs
Tuna
Anchovies
Olives
Capers
Basil
Vinaigrette (mustard, vinegar, olive oil, salt and pepper)

Mix ingredients and serve

Caprese Salad

Sliced tomatoes
Sliced mozzarella
Fresh basil leaves
Balsamic vinegar and Olive oil
Salt and pepper

Mix ingredients and serve

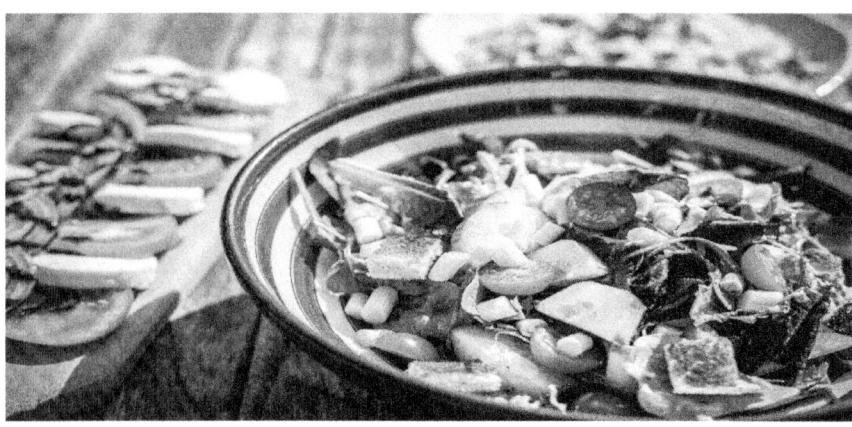

Guacamole

Avocado
Chopped tomatoes, seeds removed
Diced red onion
Juice of half a lemon or lime
Fresh coriander
Salt and pepper

Mash avocado, mix in other ingredients and serve with crudités

Hummus

Chickpeas
A clove of garlic
Juice of half a lemon
2 tablespoons of olive oil
1 teaspoon of tahini (optional)

Mix all the ingredients together in a blender and serve with crudités

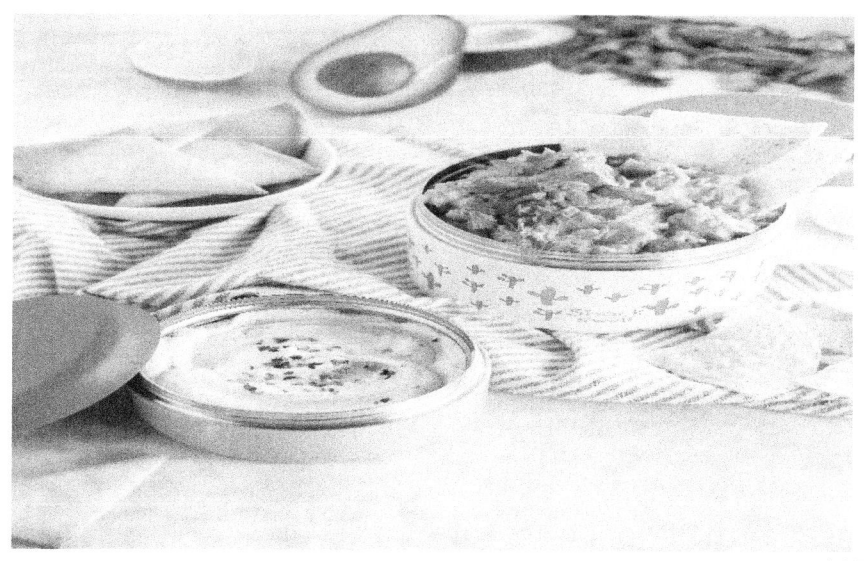

Chicken Goujons

Chicken breasts sliced into fingers
1 egg
Breadcrumbs
Salt and pepper

1. Preheat the oven to 190C;
2. Beat the egg;
3. Dip the chicken in the egg;
4. Roll the egg-soaked chicken in the breadcrumbs, having seasoned the breadcrumbs with salt and pepper;
5. Place on a greaseproof tray;
6. Drizzle with olive oil;
7. Cook in the oven for 30-40 minutes, turning over once until golden brown all over;
8. Serve with salad.

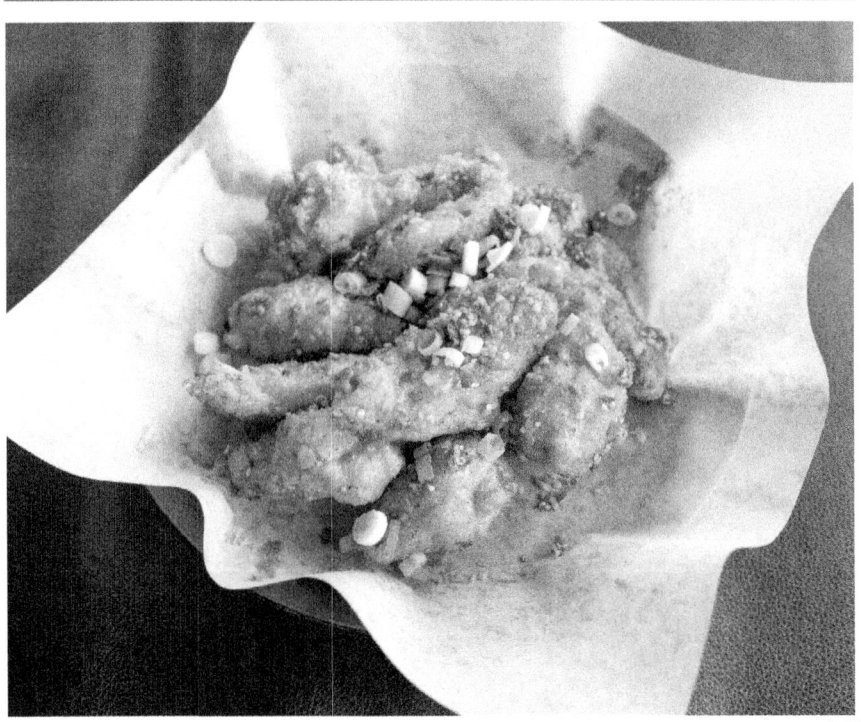

Cheese and spinach omelette

4 eggs
60g grated parmesan
300g spinach
1 chopped clove of garlic
3 spring onions

1. Heat up some olive oil in a saucepan and add the garlic, spring onions and spinach.
2. Cook until the spinach has wilted and then set aside.
3. Heat up some olive oil in a saucepan and, after whisking up the eggs with a little salt and pepper, add them to the pan and cook.
4. As the omelette is starting to set underneath, sprinkle on the parmesan.
5. As the omelette sets on top, pour the spinach mix onto half of the surface of the omelette and then fold the other half over.
6. Serve with salad on the side.

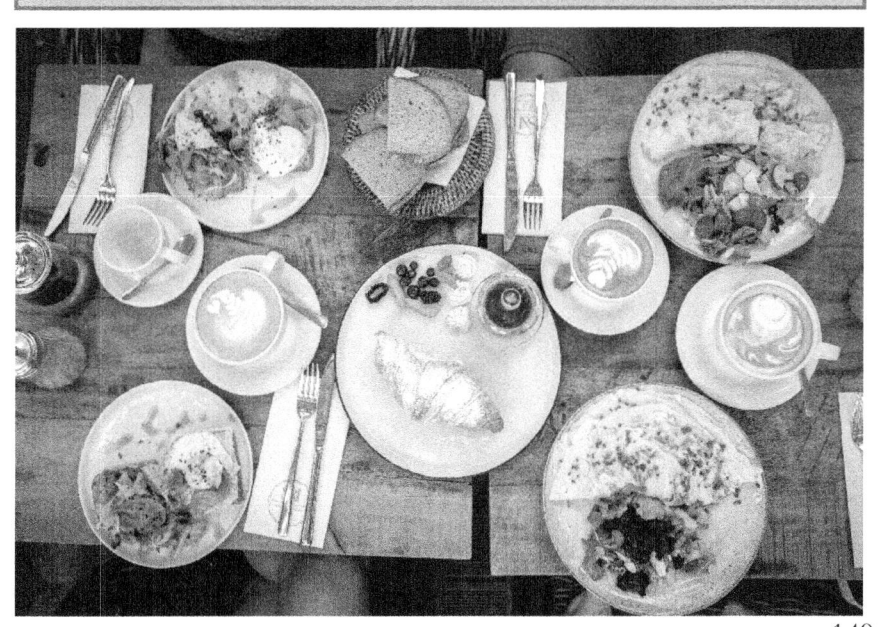

Lentil soup

400g Lentils
400g Mixed vegetables
1 onion
Turmeric, salt and pepper

1. Chop up the onion and fry it gently in some olive oil;
2. Add the vegetables and the lentils and stir together;
3. Add enough water to cover the ingredients, stir in the seasoning and bring to a gentle boil;
4. Cook for 40-45 minutes.

Red Lentil Soup

1 onion
5 large carrots
1 cup of red lentils
Turmeric, salt, pepper and fresh coriander to season

1. Chop up the onion and fry it gently in some olive oil;
2. Add the lentils and the chopped carrots, cover with water, stir in the seasoning and bring to a boil;
3. Cover saucepan and cook gently for 20-30 minutes;
4. Puree and season with coriander to serve.

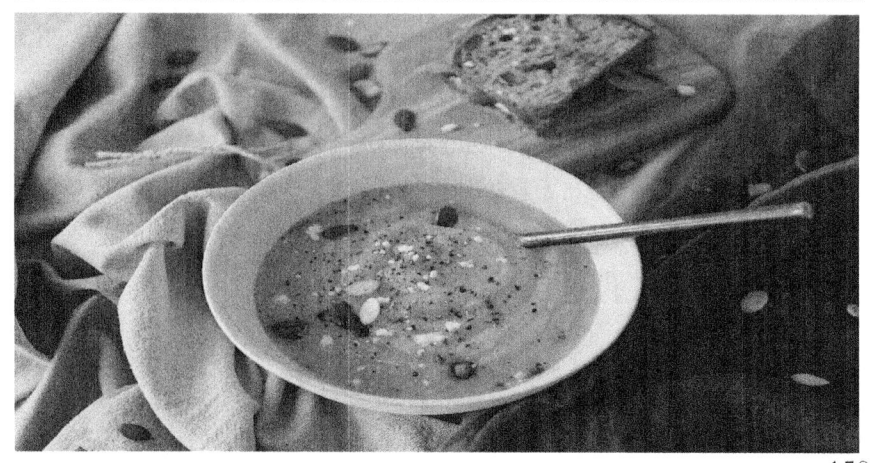

Sardines with cherry tomatoes

Sardines
Juice of half a lemon and a clove of garlic
Cherry tomatoes, quartered
Pine nuts and Fresh basil

1. Preheat the oven to 160C.
2. Line a baking tray with baking paper and place the sardines on the paper.
3. Mix the lemon juice with some olive oil and garlic and brush over the sardines before placing in the oven.
4. Mix the tomatoes, pine nuts and basil with a little olive oil and pour over the sardines once they have been cooking for 10 minutes and cook for another 3 minutes.
5. Serve with salad, brown rice or vegetables.

Salmon with cherry tomatoes and asparagus

4 salmon fillets
Juice of half a lemon and a clove of garlic
Pine nuts and Fresh basil
Cherry tomatoes and Asparagus

Cook on a bed of asparagus as above for 25 minutes.

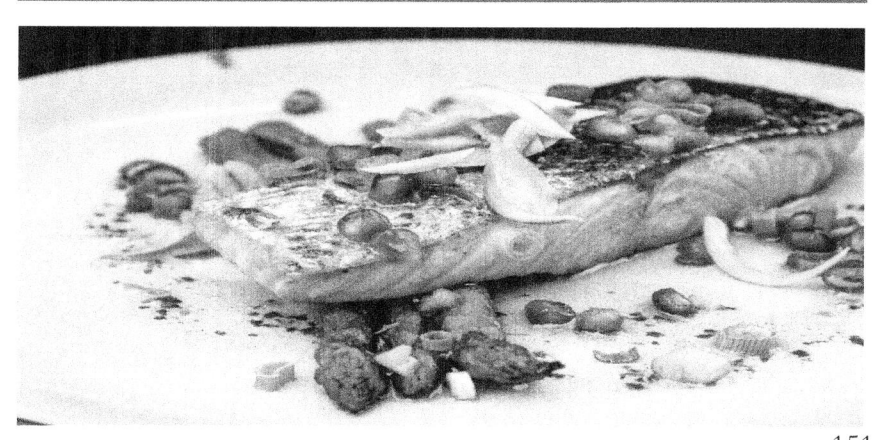

Gumbo Soup

1 cup of chopped spring onions
1 cup of diced celery and diced red pepper
2 cups of mangetout and baby corns
1 cup of chopped broccoli florets
1 cup of diced tomatoes
200g Shelled Prawns
Juice of 1 lemon or lime
Salt, pepper, ginger, turmeric, paprika and cayenne pepper
Fresh coriander

1. Fry the onions, celery and red pepper in a little olive oil;
2. Add all the other ingredients, cover with water and bring to the boil; then reduce heat and cook for 30 minutes;
3. Sprinkle with coriander to serve.

Coconut Chickpea Soup

1 onion
Mixed vegetables (carrots, cauliflower, courgettes, broccoli)
400g Chickpeas
Coconut milk
Turmeric, salt and pepper to season
Fresh coriander

1. Gently fry the onions in a little olive oil;
2. Add the mixed vegetables and the chickpeas, cover with water and bring to a gentle boil for 30 minutes;
3. Add coconut milk and sprinkle with coriander to serve.

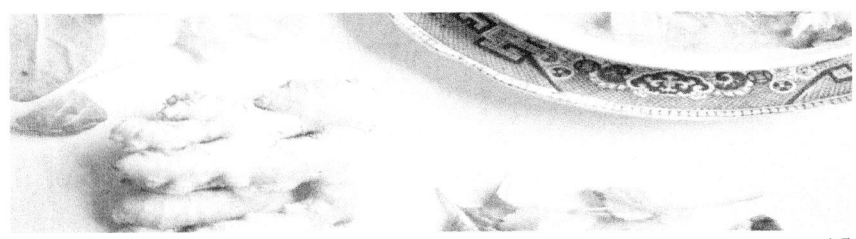

Super-Easy Pasta al Pomodoro

3 cups of chopped cherry tomatoes
2 cloves of garlic
1 teaspoon of salt
250g pasta
Fresh basil
Grana padana or parmesan cheese

1. Gently fry the tomatoes and garlic in olive oil until soft.
2. Add the salt and continue to simmer;
3. Cook the pasta in a pan of boiling water for the time required;
4. Drain the pasta and add to the saucepan of tomatoes and stir in some fresh basil until the pasta is well covered in sauce;
5. Serve with a generous sprinkling of grana padana or parmesan.

Pasta is a great go-to meal as long as it is balanced with a good source of protein. This dish can be made with meat or fish, such as anchovies or sardines in the sauce. You can also boil some vegetables, such as cauliflower and broccoli with the pasta and then, once drained, just toss over the heat for a few minutes in some olive oil and garlic and sprinkle with grana or parmesan. What is life without a plate of spaghetti every now and then?

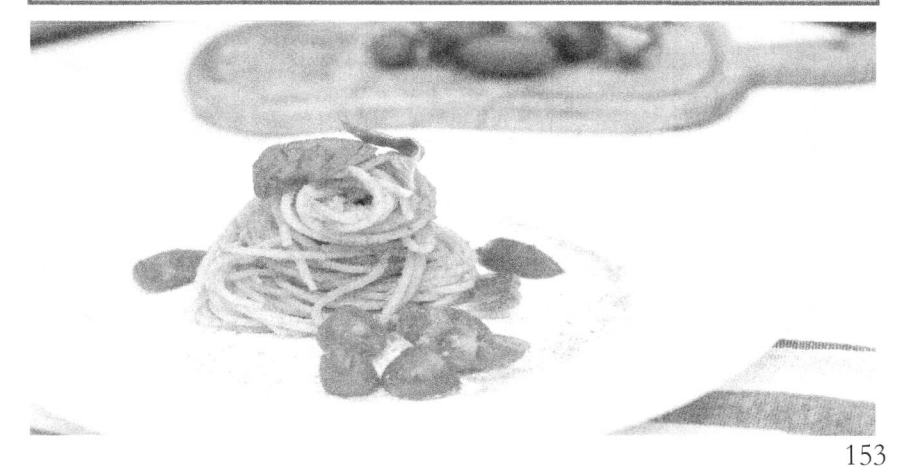

Tagliatelle al Salmone

1 onion
½ cup of peas
2 fillets of salmon
½ cup of cream
250g tagliatelle pasta

1. Gently fry the onion in olive oil until soft. And then mix in the peas
2. Add the filets of salmon, cook through and separate into chunks or flakes;
3. Season with salt and pepper (and turmeric for a yellow punch)
4. Add the cream and simmer gently;
5. Cook the pasta in a pan of boiling water for the time required;
6. Drain the pasta and add to the salmon sauce;
7. Stir in well until all the pasta is coated in sauce;
8. Serve with a sprinkle of chopped parsley.

If you prefer, you can replace the cream with a tomato sauce as per the previous recipe and add fresh basil to serve.

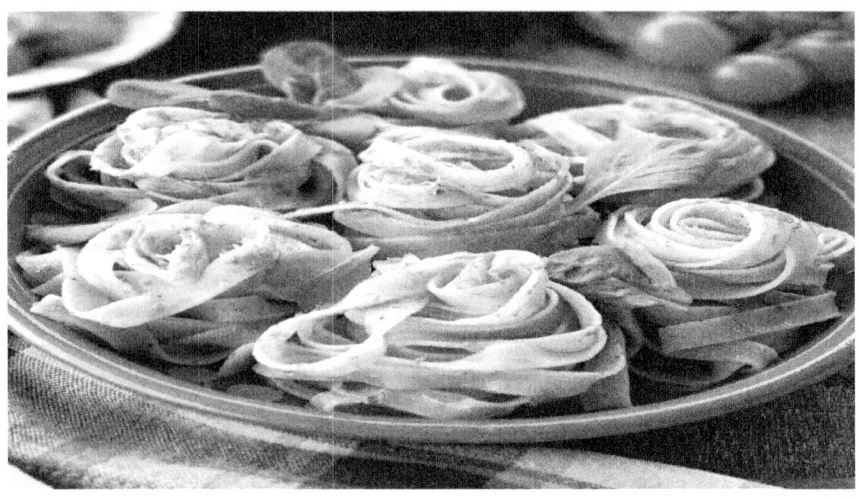

Tagliata

Filet steak

1. Slice the steak thinly and season with olive oil, salt and pepper;
2. Heat up a pan or griddle and sear the steak until cooked to your point of preference;
3. Serve on a bed of rocket salad, with flakes of grana/parmesan, balsamic vinegar and mustard.

This dish also works well with the side dishes below.

Satay Green Beans

500g Green beans
3 cloves of garlic
2 tablespoons of mustard
1 tablespoon of maple syrup or honey
1 tablespoon of peanut butter

1. Boil beans for 5 minutes, then drain;
2. Fry the diced garlic in olive oil for a few minutes before adding the drained beans;
3. Mix the other ingredients in a bowl;
4. Add the beans and garlic and mix well before serving.

Roast vegetable tray

400g potatoes & 400g cauliflower
3 cloves of garlic, turmeric, salt and pepper

1. Chop up the potatoes and cauliflower and spread on a baking tray;
2. Douse with olive oil and season with chopped garlic, turmeric, salt and pepper;
3. Roast for 45-50 minutes until crisp.

Thai Curry

Mangetout
Baby corn
Broccoli florets
Coconut milk
Chicken breast cut in squares or shelled prawns
4 cloves of garlic
Ginger, turmeric and lemongrass
Juice of 1 lime
Thai basil or fresh coriander

1. Gently fry all the seasoning (garlic, ginger, turmeric, lemongrass, salt, and pepper) in coconut oil;
2. Add the chicken or prawns and braze lightly;
3. Add the vegetables and cover with boiling water;
4. Cook for 20 minutes, then stir in the coconut milk and cook for another 5 to 10 minutes before adding the lime juice and basil or coriander.
5. Serve with rice or rice noodles.

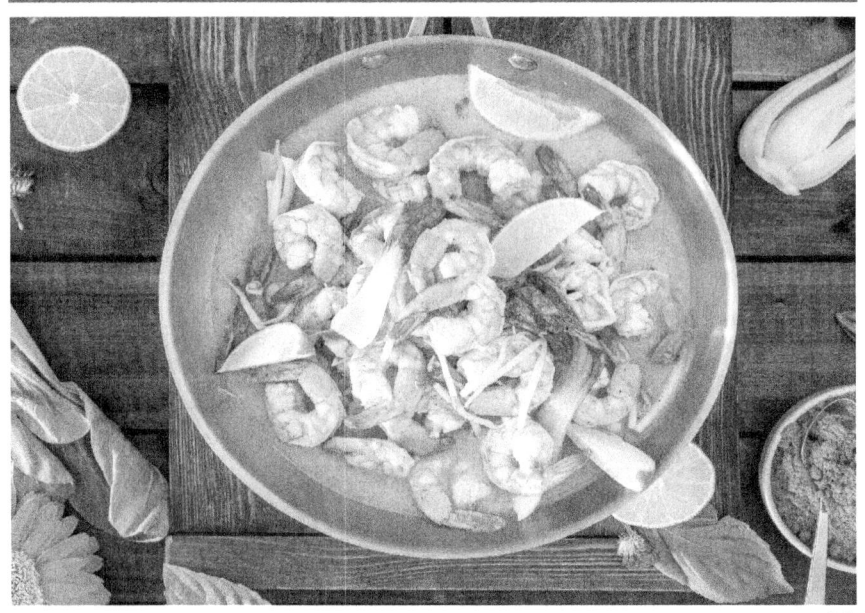

Chocolate Torte

100g ground almonds
50g cacao powder
250ml maple syrup
100g rice or oat flour
60ml chickpea water (drained from a can of chickpeas) or 2 large eggs
100g black beans or red kidney beans (rinsed and drained)
1 tablespoon of apple cider vinegar
1 tablespoon of olive oil

1. Preheat the oven to 180C;
2. Mix up all ingredients thoroughly in a large bowl;
3. Pour into a round, greaseproof-paper lined pan and cook for 25-30 minutes;
4. Remove from the pan and cool on a cooling rack.

Chocolate mousse

½ cup of pitted dates
4 Avocados
2 tablespoons of maple syrup
40g cacao powder

1. Soften dates in warm water for 10-15 minutes;
2. Blend all ingredients in a food processor until smooth;
3. Pour into individual bowls; decorate with walnuts or other nuts/seeds and cool in the fridge before serving.

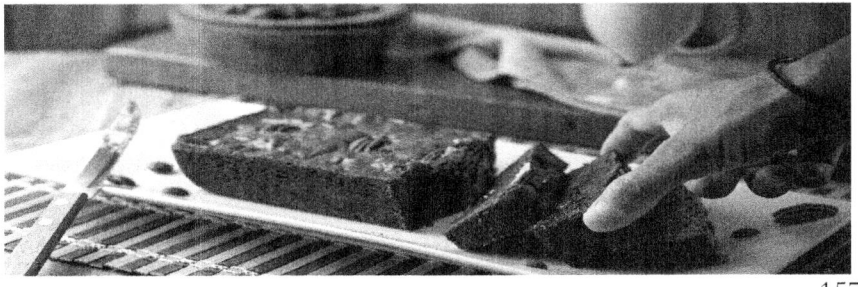

Ice Lollies

Greek yoghurt (optional)
Milk (cows, coconut, almond…)
Fruit

1. Blend your choice of fruit in a blender alone or with your choice of milk or Greek yoghurt;
2. Have fun making delicious combinations (mango and banana, pineapple and coconut milk, strawberries and Greek yoghurt…)
3. Pour into popsicle moulds and freeze for at least 5 hours.

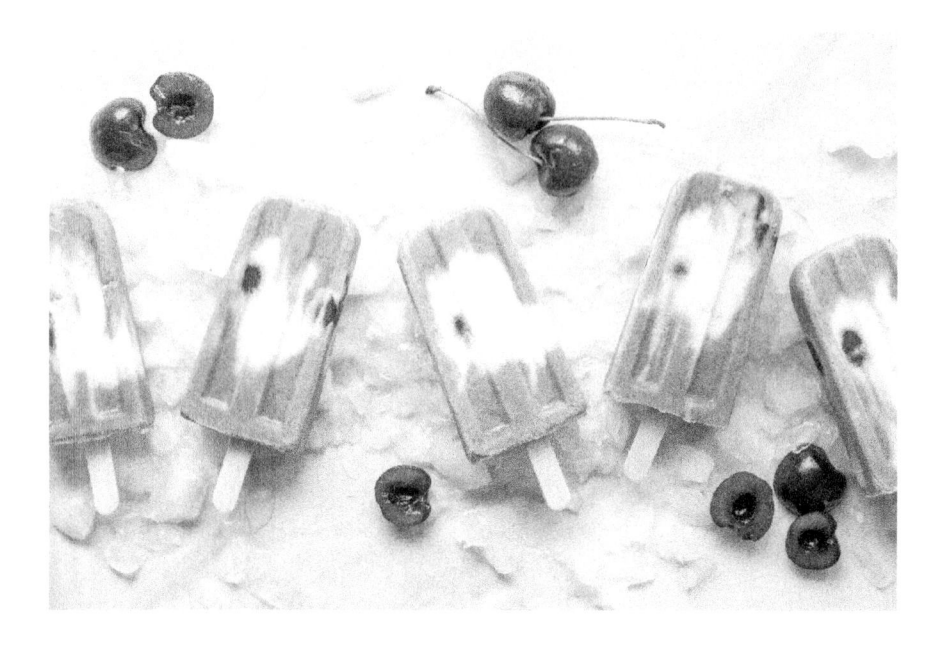

Now that we understand what to eat to optimise weight management, in the next chapter, we will explore the role of metabolism and how exercise and other tools can be used optimally to keep metabolism strong and weight management easy.

Chapter Four – METABOLISM

People commonly speak of metabolism to explain individual differences in ease of weight control or when the calorie equation doesn't add up. Some people are considered to have a fast metabolism, which allows them to eat whatever they want and still remain slim, while others have a slow metabolism and struggle to keep weight off. This use of the term metabolism actually refers to the basal metabolic rate (BMR), which if high allows and requires us to consume more energy before any excess is stored as fat. If, on the other hand, your basal metabolic rate is low, your energy requirements will be lower and can be satisfied with a lower food intake.

The basal metabolic rate is an important factor of weight management and one that, with ordinary calorie-restricted diets, can trip us up and render futile all our attempts at weight loss. In this chapter we will be exploring energy consumption and the basal metabolic rate. If you would like to learn more about this topic, continue reading. If, on the other hand, you want to jump straight into applying the tools to strengthen your basal metabolic rate, go straight to the section at the end of this chapter entitled **"METABOLISM PROTOCOL"**.

Basal Metabolic Rate (BMR)
The rate at which the body utilises energy in order to keep basic processes functioning at rest is known as the Basal Metabolic Rate (BMR). These basic processes include breathing, contraction of muscles, brain and nerve function, liver function, blood circulation, regulation of body temperature and cell growth. Your BMR makes up 60 to 75% of the body's total daily caloric expenditure depending upon level of activity. Approximately another 10% of the body's total energy expenditure is used in digestion.

Changes in BMR thwart the mathematics of many a calorie-controlled diet. Diets that restrict calories slow down the BMR because the body registers the reduction in food intake as a signal of starvation and attempts to preserve energy. As BMR falls in response to reduced calorie intake, dieters will begin to feel tired, less motivated to exercise, they will also experience heightened cold sensitivity and a dampened mood. This reaction is the bane of many a dieter's life; just as they are deploying all their willpower to restrict their food intake and increase their activity level, the body is working against their efforts by reducing their energy requirements. They are no longer, therefore, able to create the energy deficit required to lose weight.

> In our quest to attain and sustain an ideal weight, keeping our BMR strong and stable is an essential component of our success.

In our quest to attain and sustain an ideal weight, keeping our BMR strong and stable is an essential component of success. A high BMR means that more energy is required to cover essential physical needs and therefore a person with a high BMR can eat more than a person with a low BMR before the food consumed gets stored as fat instead of being utilised to cover energetic requirements. Total energetic requirements also depend

160

upon levels of activity, but the bulk of energy utilised per day is made up of the BMR. This is not an argument against physical activity, but highlights that it is difficult to depend solely upon exercise to counterbalance excess food intake. However, exercise is of vital importance to our general health and, in particular, for healthy weight management because the right kind of exercise can sustain BMR and improve our hormonal balance.

The hypothalamus is responsible for regulating the body's BMR, as well as regulating heart rate, body temperature and food intake. The following factors contribute to maintaining a strong BMR:
- A healthy thyroid;
- Lean body mass.

Thyroid health
BMR is increased by thyroid hormones triiodothyronine (T3) and thyroxine (T4) released from the thyroid gland. The synthesis of T3 and T4 is dependent upon sufficient iodine in the diet. They increase lipolysis, carbohydrate metabolism and protein turnover, therefore, favouring weight loss. Low levels of thyroid hormones result in a sluggish BMR and weight gain. Leptin resistance inhibits the effects of thyroid hormones on BMR.

Lean body mass
BMR usually decreases with age, mainly due to the fall in lean body mass common with ageing. Anaerobic exercise, in particular resistance and weight training, increases BMR by increasing muscle mass. Aerobic exercise does not generally increase muscle mass sufficiently to affect BMR. However, aerobic exercise offers many benefits for weight management, including better brain health, stress relief, better immune function and fat mobilisation.

Thermogenesis
Thermogenesis is the generation of heat in the body. Thermogenesis is a drain on energy. It can be generated through the digestion of food (with protein being the most thermogenic), through exercise,

through fidgeting known as non-exercise activity thermogenesis (NEAT) or by shivering, for example, to regulate body temperature. The body also contains some brown fat cells, which are differentiated from white fat cells as they contain mitochondria (the browner the fat, the richer in mitochondria) that use energy to generate heat. New-born babies have high levels of brown fat to help them maintain body temperature by generating heat.

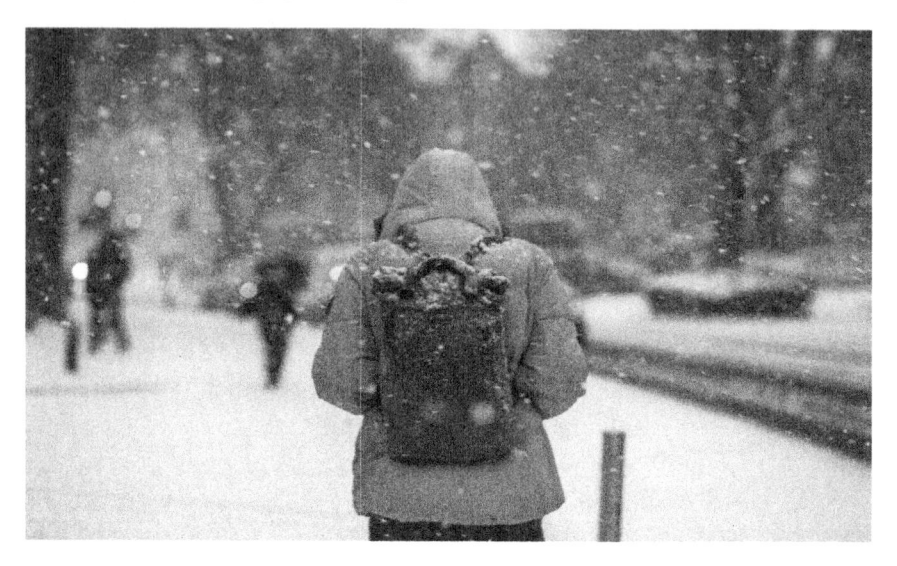

Levels of brown fat are inversely related to age, body mass index (BMI) and diabetes. The greater the total amount of fat, the less active brown fat will be.

Cold exposure has been proven to increase BMR and activate brown fat, as well as inducing mitochondrial biogenesis. However, as attractive as the prospect may be of transforming excess white fat into heat-generating, energy-consuming brown fat, it may not impact energy balance sufficiently to facilitate weight loss. This is because, as adults, we generally have such a minuscule amount of brown fat, normally an average of 10g.

However, even if brown fat or its activation does not sufficiently increase energy expenditure to cause weight loss, it does have more notable benefits. Studies show that transplanting brown fat into mice can reverse diet-induced insulin resistance and lower circulating concentrations of triglycerides, cholesterol and glucose.

> Cold exposure has been proven to increase BMR and activate brown fat, as well as inducing mitochondrial biogenesis.

Thermogenesis via brown fat is regulated by a specific protein called sLR11. A decrease in sLR11 allows for an increase in thermogenesis and a reduction in fat mass. This protein has been of importance in our evolutionary survival as it has allowed us to store fat efficiently instead of wasting it through thermogenesis unless absolutely necessary during cold exposure.

One study showed that sLR11 suppresses thermogenesis in mice and mice lacking sLR11 show increased browning of white adipose tissue, display hypermetabolism and are protected from diet-induced obesity.

In humans, sLR11 levels are positively correlated with BMI and body fat, which suggests that the energy-conserving role of sLR11 (it prevents the browning of white adipose tissue) is amplified as weight accrues. sLR11 has been shown to regulate lipoprotein lipase (LPL), facilitating fat storage, whereas the absence of sLR11 facilitated thermogenesis, reduced fat storage, increased recruitment of brown adipocytes, and drove hypermetabolism and leanness. Whether burning energy through increased adipose thermogenesis would also have the same effect in humans still needs to be established.

Some thermogenesis can be stimulated with herbal thermogenic aids, such as caffeine, berberine, guarana, ginseng, mustard seed, chilli peppers and cayenne pepper.

> Incorporating cold showers into our daily routine has been shown to have numerous benefits from reduced stress levels and greater stress resilience to an improved immune response, stronger cognitive function, better circulation, reduced inflammation and easier weight management.

Incorporating cold showers into our daily routine has been shown to have numerous benefits from reduced stress levels and greater stress resilience to an improved immune response, stronger cognitive function, better circulation, reduced inflammation and easier weight management.

Build up slowly by starting with just a few seconds of cold water in your normal shower, switching back to warm before trying a few more seconds. You will find you can build up to longer, more invigorating sessions. Many athletes enjoy the benefits of ice baths and proponents, such as Wim Hof, have espoused the practice of cold water immersion, with the adjunct of breathing and meditative exercises, as a means of controlling the autonomic nervous system, stimulating the immune response, reducing inflammation and releasing stress.

Physical Exercise
The value of physical exercise is not confined to weight management. Further benefits include cardiovascular health, immune health, bone density, digestive health, improved strength and muscular development, brain health, mental health and pure enjoyment. These benefits can be achieved with around one and a half hours of exercise a week.

Exercise is classified into three categories: aerobic, anaerobic and flexibility training. Aerobic exercise, such as running, dancing, tennis, brisk walking, swimming and cycling, is exercise that increases the body's use of oxygen while increasing the heart rate. Anaerobic exercise, such as weight training, interval training and sprints, is exercise that exceeds the oxygen threshold and promotes strength, power and endurance and develops lean body mass. Flexibility exercise, such as yoga and stretching, improves our range of movement, agility, elasticity of joints and reduces the incidence of injury.

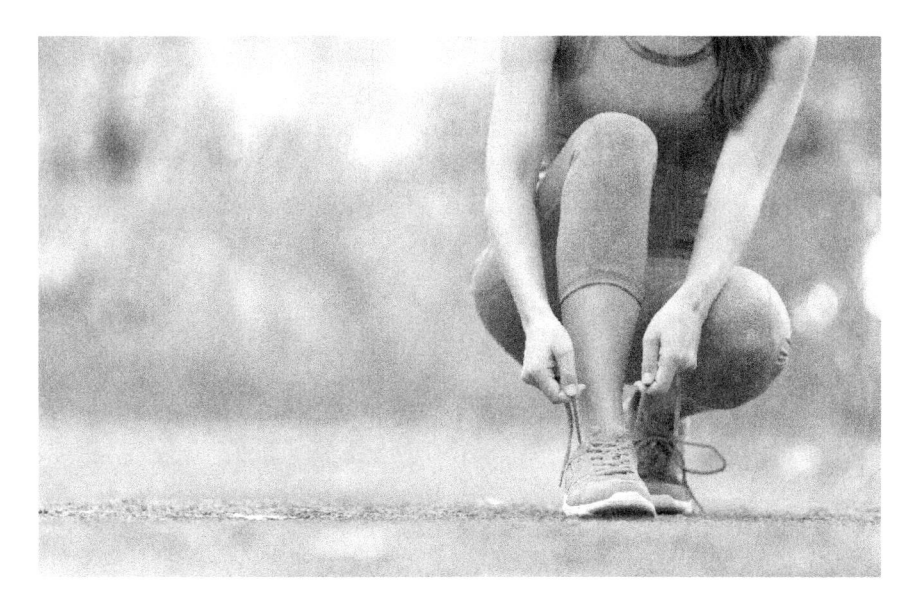

Regular exercise stimulates blood flow to fat tissue and enhances fat mobilisation, that is, the transportation of fatty acids from fat tissue to skeletal muscles for energy production. Exercise is, therefore, a vital pillar of successful weight management. Studies have shown that when obese subjects are enrolled in an aerobic exercise programme, maximal oxygen consumption (VO2max) increases, body weight and fat mass are reduced, insulin sensitivity increases while leptin levels fall slightly, reducing leptin resistance.

Aerobic exercise is any activity that stimulates the heart rate and breathing to increase, but not so much that you can't sustain the activity for more than a few minutes. Aerobic means "with oxygen," and anaerobic means "without oxygen." Anaerobic exercise is the type of exercise that gets you out of breath in just a few moments, like lifting weights, sprinting or climbing a flight of stairs.

Exercise can increase BMR through an increase in lean body mass and through the training effect. The training effect consists of at least four weeks of targeted training up to and beyond the anaerobic threshold, which is the point at which the body must switch from aerobic to anaerobic metabolism for energy production. Consistent training of this type promotes mitochondrial biogenesis, increasing mitochondrial density and allowing for increased aerobic potential. This leads to a lower resting heart rate and an increased BMR.

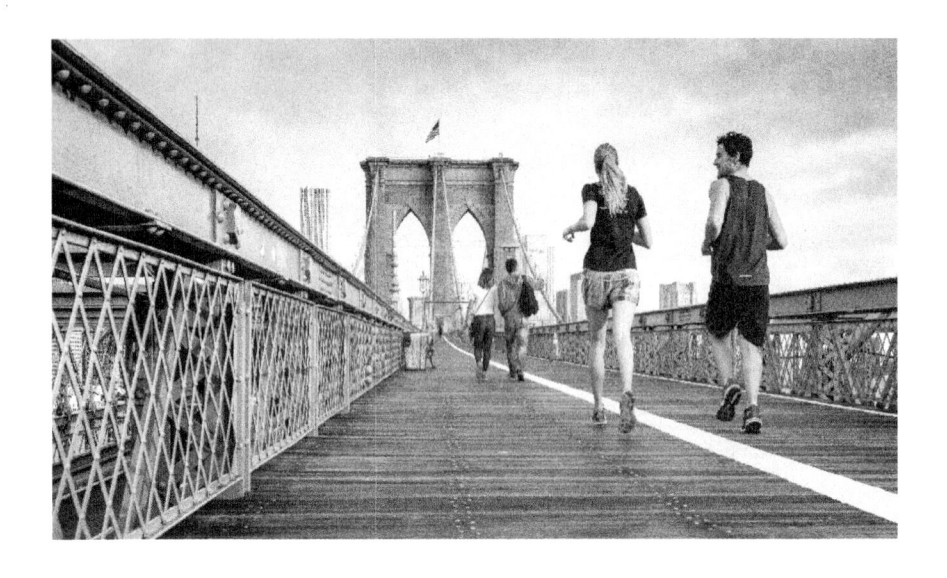

The training effect increases vital lung capacity allowing more oxygen to be delivered from the lungs into the blood. Red blood cells transport the oxygen to cells and dispose of returning waste. Aerobic training increases levels of haemoglobin, red blood cells, blood plasma and total blood volume. The result is enhanced energy production and increased endurance.

Greater muscle mass increases BMR, so weight-training that increases muscle mass can increase resting energy requirements by increasing BMR. Burst training, involving sprints and high intensity interval training, has also been shown to reduce ghrelin levels, which consequently attenuates appetite and food intake, and increases HGH levels, which strengthens muscle mass, compounding the heightened BMR effect. Studies also show that burst training induces mitochondrial biogenesis and increases blood concentrations of the soluble leptin receptor (sOB-R), therefore, even though exercise reduces leptin levels, higher sOB-R levels increase the body's sensitivity to leptin.

Furthermore, as exercise stimulates the release of endorphins and serotonin, it can attenuate the incentive salience of food intake, as well as improving mood and self-esteem. It reduces cortisol levels and also enhances cognitive function, upgrades memory, improves our ability to cope with stress and elevates markers of neurotrophic factors, such as brain-derived neurotrophic factor (BDNF). It is, therefore, beneficial for the treatment of depression.

Timing

Timing is also important when it comes to exercise. Studies have shown that exercising before eating breakfast mobilises more fat reserves, improves insulin sensitivity and increases glucose uptake into muscle tissue compared to exercising later in the day. Exercising in this fasted state also induces mitochondrial adaptations in muscle and fat tissue facilitating greater fat utilisation. Gene activity related to fatty acid metabolism increases thanks to fasted exercise such that cells become more efficient at burning fat for energy in the long-term and not just during exercise. Fasted exercise also reduces ghrelin levels

> Timing is also important when it comes to exercise. Studies have shown that exercising before eating breakfast mobilises more fat reserves compared to exercising later in the day.

thus attenuating appetite and food intake and improving fat loss and weight maintenance.

However, any form of exercise at any time of day that counterbalances our increasingly sedentary lifestyle is favourable to healthy weight management. Modern living is generally far less physically demanding than in the past; we tend to sit at desks all day and employ appliances to do tasks, such as washing our clothes, that we once had to consume energy to complete by hand. Integrating more activity into our day, such as taking the stairs instead of the lift or walking and cycling instead of using transportation, can significantly aid weight management.

Optimum Exercise
Our exercise routine should ideally include some aerobic, some anaerobic and some flexibility-enhancing exercise. Aerobic exercise optimises cardiovascular health, which means that oxygen is efficiently delivered where needed and carbon dioxide and metabolic waste products are expelled efficiently. Aerobic exercise also utilises energy and mobilises fat reserves. It also increases the number of mitochondria in skeletal muscle cells, increasing the body's ability to generate energy. Anaerobic exercise has similar benefits with the added ability to strengthen and develop muscle tissue. Flexibility exercises keep us supple.

In order to reap the optimum training effect from aerobic exercise, it is advisable to exercise at 55% to 85% of our maximum heart rate, which is calculated by subtracting our age from 220. So, at 50, a good level of aerobic training would raise your heartbeat over 94 beats per minute (bpm), but no more than 145bpm. It has been found that bursts of anaerobic exercise mixed with aerobic exercise can be highly efficient at both increasing lean body

> A combination of aerobic, anaerobic and flexibility exercise is the ideal routine for optimum health and weight management.

mass and reaping cardiovascular benefits. A combination of aerobic, anaerobic and flexibility exercise is the ideal routine for optimum health and weight management.

High Intensity Interval Training

High-intensity interval training (HIIT), also called high-intensity intermittent exercise (HIIE), is a cardiovascular exercise strategy that alternates short periods of intense anaerobic exercise with less intense recovery periods. HIIT sessions can last from a few minutes to thirty minutes, depending on the participant's level of fitness or time available.

A version of HIIT conceived by Professor Izumi Tabata of Ritsumeikan University involves 20 seconds of ultra-intense exercise followed by 10 seconds of rest, repeated continuously for 4 minutes (8 cycles). Professor Tabata found that athletes using this method exercised only 4 minutes per day compared to their usual hour-long sessions, but achieved comparable aerobic improvements with greater anaerobic capacity.

HIIT workouts are a fast and efficient way to improve physical fitness and mobilise fat reserves. HIIT significantly lowers insulin resistance compared to other forms of exercise and encourages increased weight loss compared to other methods. A study found that seven sessions of HIIT over a 2-week period improved whole body fat oxidation and increased the capacity for skeletal muscle to oxidise fat in moderately active women. A 2010 systematic review of HIIT summarised the results of HIIT on fat loss and stated that HIIT can result in notable reductions of subcutaneous fat in young and healthy individuals, and greater, more significant reductions for overweight individuals.

Use the exercises at the end of this chapter to tap into the time-efficient benefits of HIIT.

METABOLISM PROTOCOL

If you are currently doing no exercise, it is vital for your general health and successful weight management to start integrating some enjoyable movement into your day. Start with an easy walk. Go somewhere beautiful in nature. Making the exercise experience an enjoyable part of your day that you look forward to is crucial in order to consistently integrate it into your routine. You will want to do it, rather than forcing yourself to do it.

The following steps will contribute to strengthening your BMR, making exercise an enjoyable addition to your daily routine, developing strength and agility, giving you greater body confidence and enhancing your quality of life.

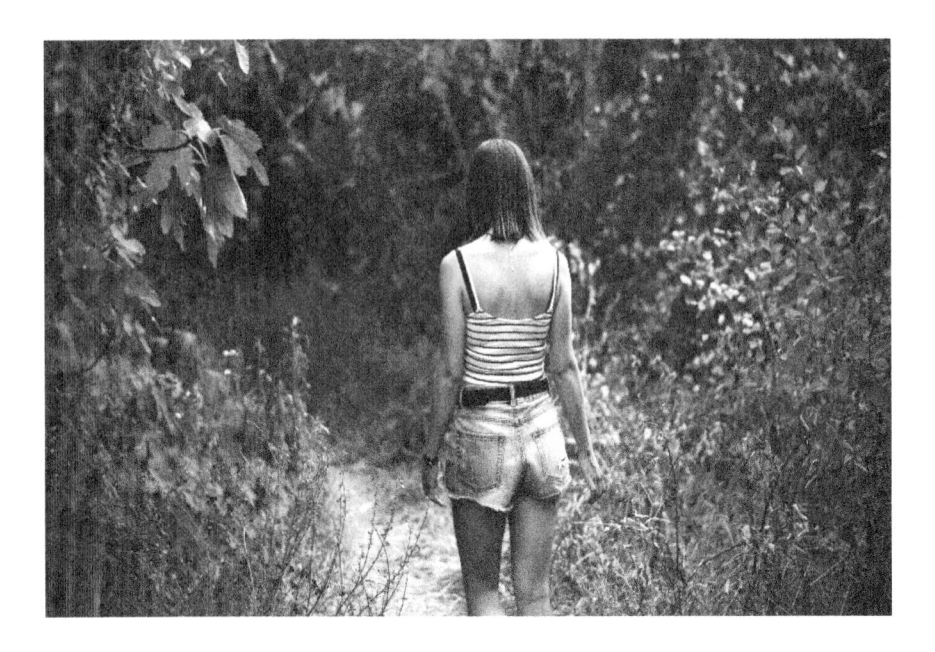

Step One: Dietary Considerations

A healthy thyroid depends upon sufficient iodine in your diet. If your diet is deficient in iodine, consider an iodine supplement or an iodine-rich botanical, such as kelp.

Make sure that your diet contains sufficient protein. Around 0.8g of protein per kilogram of weight should be sufficient unless you are training beyond the parameters of this protocol. Isolated amino acids, such as arginine, glutamine and lysine, have been found to enhance the release of human growth hormone from the pituitary gland thus supporting lean body mass, facilitating weight management and improving recovery.

Therefore, the following supplements are recommended:
- ✓ Kelp
- ✓ Arginine, Glutamine and Lysine
- ✓ A protein shake (if you struggle to integrate sufficient protein from your diet).

Step Two: Cold Exposure
Cold exposure can increase energy expenditure and strengthen your BMR. Use the following methods to integrate cold exposure into your day:

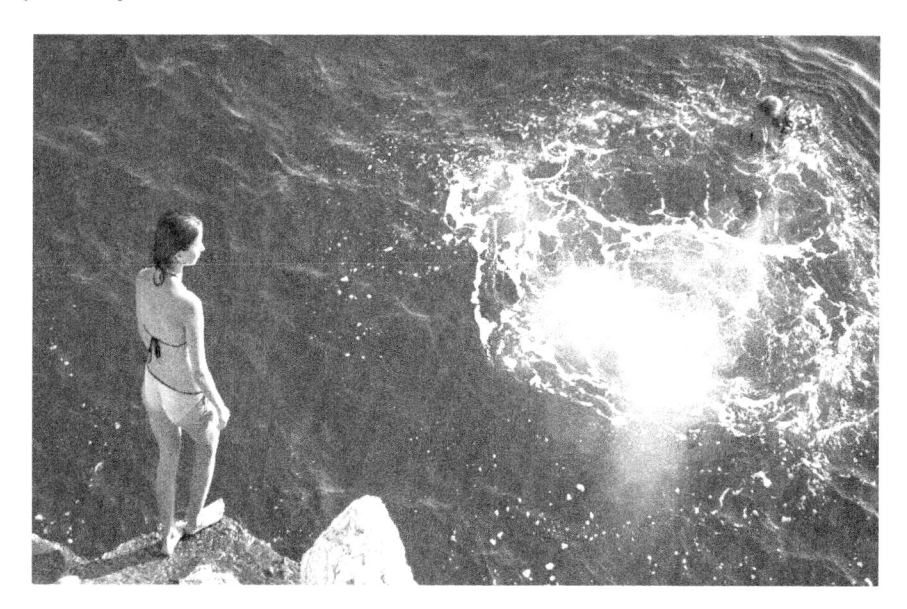

- ✓ Experiment with a few seconds under a cold shower. Try to build up to 20 seconds, each time alternating with warm water.
- ✓ Immerse as much of your body as you can stand in cold water, take a cold bath, an ice bath or go for dips in the sea, in lakes or rivers.
- ✓ Reduce the thermostat to 20 degrees centigrade in winter.

Step Three: Your Exercise Routine
Once you have introduced movement into your day and have a regular exercise practice (maybe you have started walking daily in your lunch hour), start to integrate some strength-training exercises into your routine (pick a few exercises from the list below) and always remember a few stretches to finish. The key to this stage is to start enjoying exercise and to start feeling the benefits in terms of improved mood, higher self-esteem and easier weight management. Stay at this stage until you feel the urge to expand and improve your fitness level.

The aim is to have a daily practice structured as below with a warm up, a sustained workout and a cool down with stretching:

Warm Up
Rotate joints (ankles, knees, pelvis, torso, arms, wrists and neck)
Marching or jogging on the spot for a couple of minutes

Workout
Aerobic exercise (walking, swimming, cycling, dancing, rowing, etc.)
High-intensity interval training (HIIT)

Cool Down
Slow march on the spot or walk
Stretching

The above wokout combines aerobic with anaerobic exercise along with flexibility exercises. It can be adapted according to your fitness level. So, an example of a beginner's routine would be a warm-up involving rotating the joints, followed by a 15- to 20-minute walk, some lunges, crunches and tricep dips, followed by some gentle stretches. A more advanced version would involve a warm-up, rotating the joints and jogging on the spot, followed by a 20-minute run and 3 circuits of the HIIT exercises listed below, with 15 minutes of stretching or yoga to finish.

HIIT Exercises
In order to put together a balanced routine for the HIIT section of your workout, choose one exercise per day from each section below. Start with 10 repetitions and build up to 30 or more depending on the exercise. As your fitness level improves, increase the number of exercises you complete to ten, making sure you take at least one from each section, or you can repeat the sequence of seven exercises twice or more times. You can also use the tabata method of completing the maximum number of repetitions in 20 or 30 seconds, followed by a 10- to 15-second break before continuing to the next exercise.

In the space of a week, try to complete all 7 exercises from each section, or at least 5, as each section targets a different set of muscles and each exercise in each section engages the targeted muscles in a different way. So, you could follow the sequence suggested taking the number one exercise from each section to make up your Monday workout (see below), take the number two exercise from each section for your Tuesday workout and so on, so that, in the space of a week, you will complete all seven exercises from each section.

Example of your Monday workout:
1. Plank Jack
2. Tricep Dips
3. Squats
4. Jumping Jacks
5. Glute Bridge

6. Elbow to Knee Crunches
7. Flutter Kicks

Sections 1 and 2 are for upper body strength, sections 3, 4 and 5 are to tone and develop the leg and glute muscles, and sections 6 and 7 are for torso strength, including developing the abdominal muscles for that much-desired six-pack.

Upper Body Exercises
Section 1
1. Plank Jack
   Start in a plank position with either your elbows or hands directly below your shoulders, jump your feet out wide to the sides like a jumping jack and back together again. Repeat.

2. Plank to downward dog
   Start in a plank position with either your elbows or hands on the floor directly below your shoulders. Push back into a

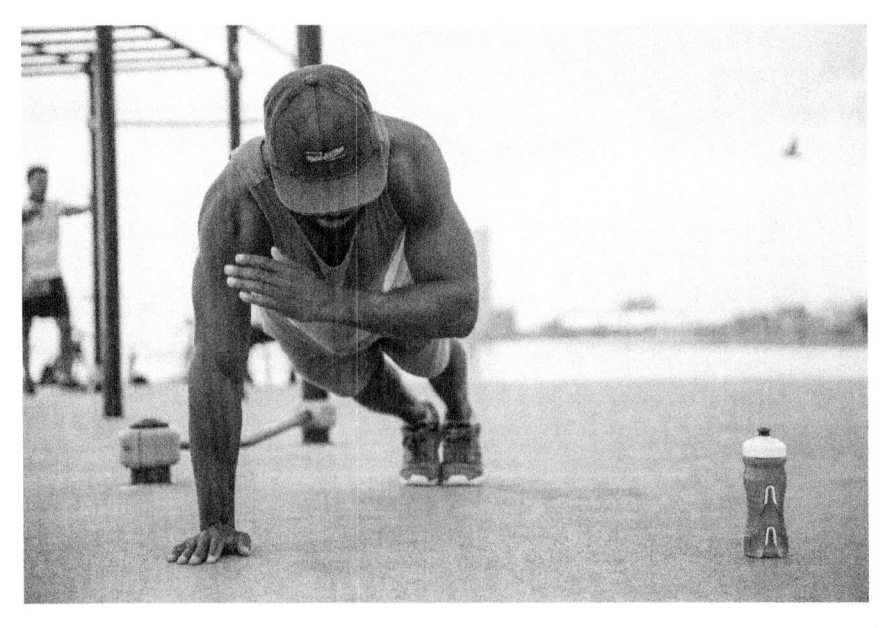

downward dog position without moving the position of your hands/elbows. Return to your starting position. Repeat.

3. Lateral plank walk
   Start in a plank position. Simultaneously step your left foot and left hand to the left. Follow with your right foot and right hand. Then, step your right foot and hand to the right, followed by your left foot and hand, so that you are back in your starting position. Repeat.

4. Plank with shoulder taps
   Start in a high plank position. Keeping your hips square to the floor, lift your right hand and tap your left shoulder. Return to the starting position and repeat with the other arm.

5. Plank to push up
   Start in a high plank position with your hands directly underneath your shoulders and your core muscles engaged. Lift one arm up and place your elbow down, followed by the other arm, so you are now on your elbows. Return to the

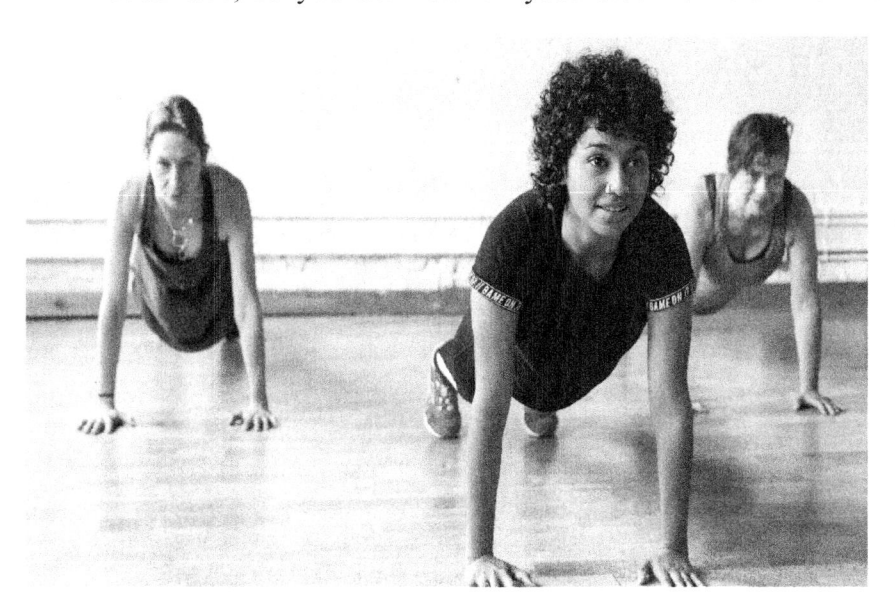

starting position by lifting one elbow up at a time and placing your hands back in the original position, until you are back to a high plank position. Repeat.

6. Plank with arm extensions
Starting in a high plank position, reach one arm out to the front in line with your body. Return to the floor and repeat on the other side. In order to increase the level of difficulty, you can try lifting your opposite leg at the same time as your arm.

7. Straight Plank
Starting in a high plank or on your elbows, engage your abs and glutes and hold for 30 seconds. As your level of fitness improves, you can hold for 60 seconds.

Section 2

1. Tricep Dips
From the crab position or off the edge of a bench, knees bent at a 90-degree angle, feet planted on the floor and hands either side of your hips, lower your body a few inches by bending your elbows and then raise your body back to the starting position.

2. Bicep Curls
Stand with feet shoulder-width apart. With your palms facing forward and holding weights, bend your elbows and pull the weights up towards your shoulders and then lower. Repeat

3. Push-ups
Start in the high plank position with your hands slightly wider than shoulder-width apart (you can also do these with your knees on the floor). Bend your elbows and lower your chest towards the floor until you are about 10-15cm away from touching the floor with your body, then push on your hands to return to the starting position. Repeat.

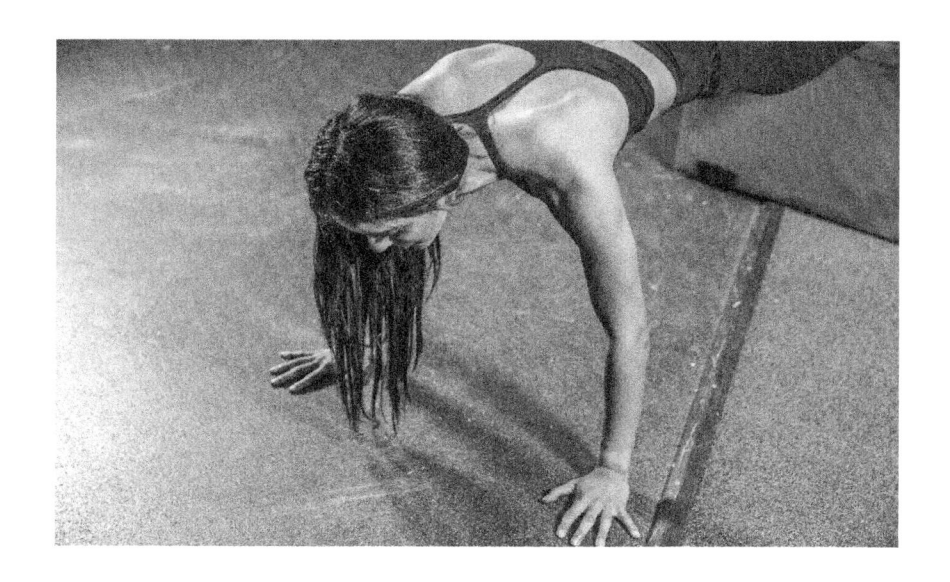

4. Punch ball
   Standing with one foot forward, hold your fists up to an imaginary punch ball. Rotate your fists as if you were punching the ball. Repeat on the other side with your other foot forward.

5. Rotate with weights (arms outstretched)
   Stand tall with your knees slightly bent and your feet hip-width apart. Holding a weight in each hand, raise your arms out to the sides until they are level with your shoulders. Make small circles with your hands, keeping your arms straight and out to the sides. Rotate first forwards and then backwards.

6. Superman with arm rotation
   Start by lying on your stomach with your arms extended forward and your legs straight. Raise all four limbs, your head and chest off the floor. Swing your arms out wide and back to touch your sides and then circle them back to the starting position. Repeat.

7. Arm lifts
   Stand tall with your knees slightly bent and your feet hip-width apart. Holding a weight in each hand, raise your weights above your head until your arms are straight above your shoulders. Bend your elbows to bring the weights back down to your shoulders then repeat.

Legs and Glutes
Section 3
1. Squats
   Stand with your feet hip-width apart and your feet pointing slightly outwards. Bend your knees, pushing your glutes out behind you so that your knees don't protrude over your feet and your thighs are parallel to the floor. Rise up, squeezing your glutes forward as you straighten. Repeat.
2. Lunges

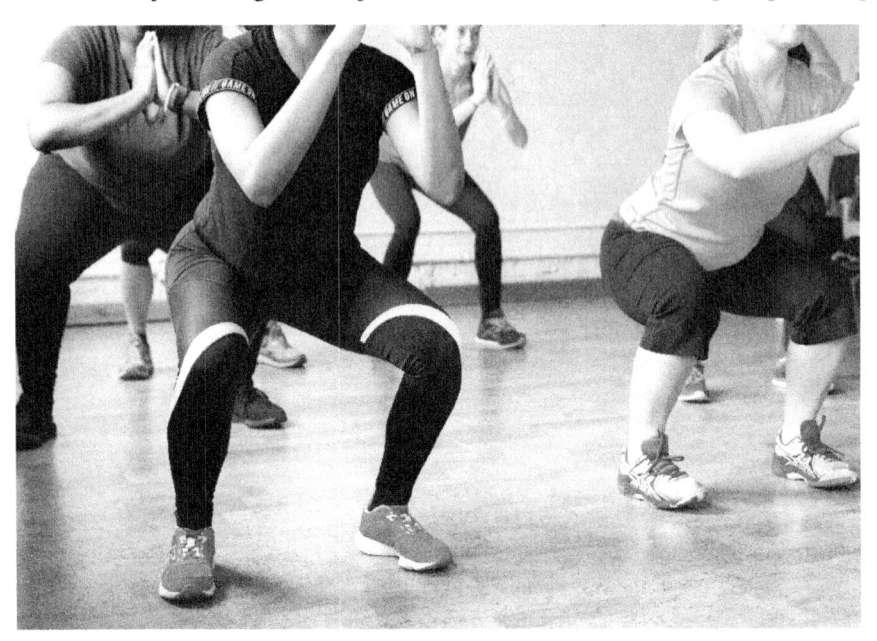

Stand tall with your feet hip-width apart. Engage your core. Take a big step forward with your right foot, shifting your weight forward so that your heel hits the floor first. Lower your body until your right thigh is parallel to the floor and your right shin is vertical. You can lightly tap your left knee to the floor, before returning to the starting position. Repeat on the other side.

3. Reverse lunges
   Stand tall with your feet hip-width apart. Engage your core. Take a big step backward with right foot. Lower your body until your left thigh is parallel to the floor and your left shin is vertical. You can lightly tap your right knee to the floor, before returning to the starting position. Repeat on the other side.

4. Side lunges
   Stand with your legs slightly wider than shoulder-distance apart and your toes pointed forward. Step to the right bending your right knee until it reaches a 90-degree angle and the other leg is straight. Press your glutes back behind you. Return to your starting position and repeat on the other side.

5. 30 Plies with 30 pulses
   Stand with your feet wider than your shoulders and turned out so that your inner thighs face forward, with your hands clasped in front of chest. Tuck your pelvis under and lower down into a wide-legged squat aiming to get your thighs parallel to the floor. Return to the starting position and repeat. On the last repetition, pulse in the lower position for an extra 10/20/30.

6. Forward leg lifts
   Stand with your legs together, shift your weight onto your left leg and extend your arms out to the side for balance. Lift your

right leg up in front of your body keeping it straight. Return to the starting position and repeat on the other side.

7. Backward leg lifts
Stand with your legs together, shift your weight onto your left leg and extend your left arm out to the side for balance. Reach down to the floor with your right arm, bending forward with your body and lifting your right leg straight back behind your body until your leg and body are parallel to the floor. Return to the starting position and repeat on the other side.

Section 4

1. Jumping Jacks
Stand tall with your feet together and your arms by your sides. Jump both feet out to the side and at the same time bring your arms above your head into a star position. Jump your feet back into the starting position and bring your arms back to your sides at the same time. Repeat.

2. Karate kicks
Stand tall with feet hip-width apart. Engage your core. Shift your weight onto your left leg and lift your right foot off the

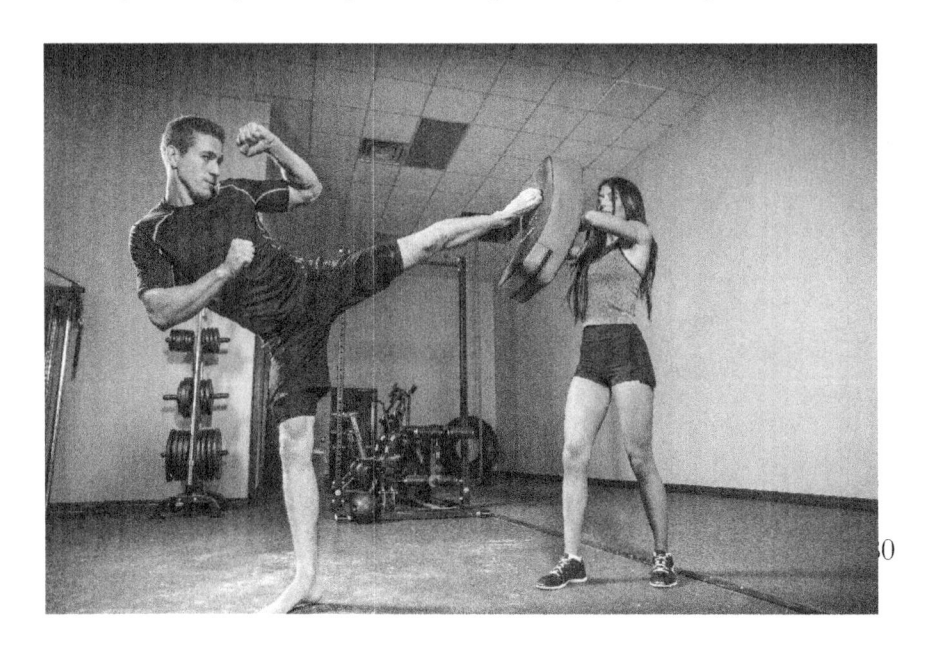

floor. Look over your right shoulder and, holding your arms up for balance, kick your right leg back as high as possible without losing balance. Lower it back to the floor before repeating for 10/20/30 repetitions. Repeat on the other side for the same number of repetitions.

3. Squat kicks
Start in a squat position with your feet slightly wider than your shoulders, your thighs parallel to the floor and your hands clasped in front of your chest. Rise up and kick one leg out to the front, before returning to the starting position and repeating on the other side.

4. Squat jumps
Start in a squat with your feet slightly wider than your shoulders, your thighs parallel to floor. Touch the floor, then jump and reach up with both arms into the air. Return down to the starting position and repeat.

5. Burpee Squats
Start in a high plank position with your feet mat-width apart. Jump your feet forward behind your hands and, then quickly lift your torso up while lowering your glutes toward floor, into a squat position. Hold the squat for a couple of seconds before placing your hands back down on the floor and jumping your feet back into the starting plank position. Repeat.

6. Speed Skater
Stand with your feet hip-width apart. Take a big step or a hop out to the right and, as you do, sweep your left leg behind you while bringing your left arm across your body and your right arm out to the side. Then, step or hop to the left, bringing your right leg behind you and your right arm across your body with your left arm out to the side. Continue alternating sides while building up speed.

7. Mountain climber
   Start in a high plank position with your feet hip-width apart. Jump your right foot in towards your hands by bending your right knee, then switch, extending your right foot back to where it started and simultaneously bringing your left foot up towards your hands by bending your left knee. Alternate legs as fast as you can.

Section 5
1. Glute bridge
   Lie on your back with your legs bent and your feet flat on the floor. Squeeze your glutes and lift your hips off the floor until your body forms one straight line from your shoulders to your knees. Hold for a few seconds before returning to the starting position. For extra strength, when you have completed your repetitions, pulse 10/20/30 times in the high position.

2. Side Leg Lifts
   Lie down on a mat on your right side with your feet stacked one on top of the other. Hold your head up with your right hand, elbow on the mat, and place your left hand on the floor in front of your torso for support. Engage your leg and glute muscles as you raise your left leg up to the side. Lower to the starting position. Repeat for 10/20/30 repetitions before completing the same number of repetitions on the other side.

3. Inner Thigh Lifts
   Lie down on a mat on your right side with your feet stacked one on top of the other. Hold your head up with your right hand, elbow on the mat, and place your left hand on the floor in front of your torso for support. Bend your left knee and place it on the floor in front of your hips. Engage your right leg muscles and lift your right leg off the floor, keeping it straight and long. Lower to the starting position. Repeat for 10/20/30 repetitions before completing the same number of repetitions on the other side.

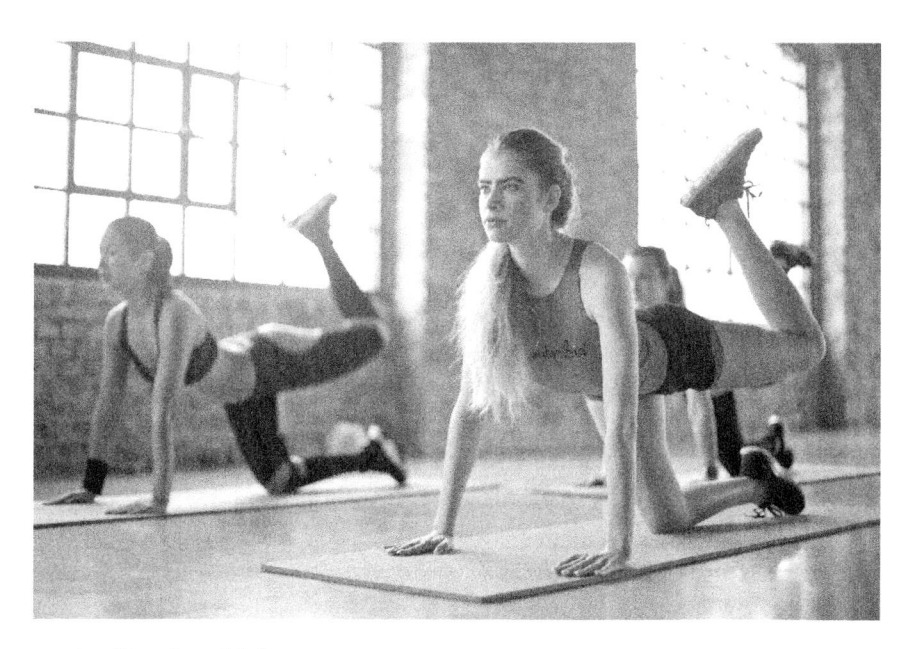

4. Donkey kicks
   Start on all fours on the floor with your wrists directly under your shoulders and your knees under your hips. Keeping your hips level and right leg bent at 90 degrees, lift your right foot upwards until your thigh is parallel to floor. Then return to the starting position. Repeat 10/20/30 times and then complete the same number of repetitions on the left side.

5. Wide-leg glute bridge
   Lie on your back with your legs bent and your feet flat on the floor, mat-width apart and slightly turned out. Squeeze your glutes and lift your hips off the floor until your body forms one straight line from your shoulders to your knees. Hold for a few seconds before returning to the starting position. For extra strength, when you have completed your repetitions, pulse 10/20/30 times in the high position.

6. Side donkey lifts
   Start on all fours on the floor with your wrists under your shoulders and your knees under your hips. Keeping your hips

level and your right leg bent at a 90-degree angle, lift your right knee out to side until your thigh is parallel to the floor. Return to the starting position. Repeat 10/20/30 times and then complete the same number of repetitions on the left side.

7. Seated to glute bridge
   Sit on the floor with your legs extended straight out in front of you. Place your palms on the floor at your sides, fingers facing forward. Straighten your back. Lift up your glutes, placing your weight on your heels. Lift your head back into a bridge position with your body in a straight line from your neck to your knees. Let your glutes lower back into the starting position. Repeat.

Abs
Section 6

1. Elbow to Knee Crunches
   Lie flat on your back and place your hands behind your head. Bend your knees and bring them up off the floor so that your thighs and hips form a 90-degree angle, calves parallel to the floor. Twist your upper body, bringing your elbow to the opposite knee while fully extending your other leg. Hold and then return back to the starting position to repeat on the other side.

2. Heel taps
   Lie down on your mat with your lower back pressed into the floor, your feet flat and shoulder-width apart and your knees bent. Raise your head and shoulders off the floor, looking between your legs. Reach your right arm down the right side of your body to touch your right heel. Repeat on your left side. Alternate touching each heel by moving from side to side, keeping your head and shoulders raised off the floor.

3. Russian Twists
   Sit on the floor and hold your legs out straight off the floor. Engage your core and lean back slightly so that your torso and legs form a V-like shape. Balancing in this position, twist your torso from side to side without moving your legs. You can hold a weight as you twist for extra strengthening potential.

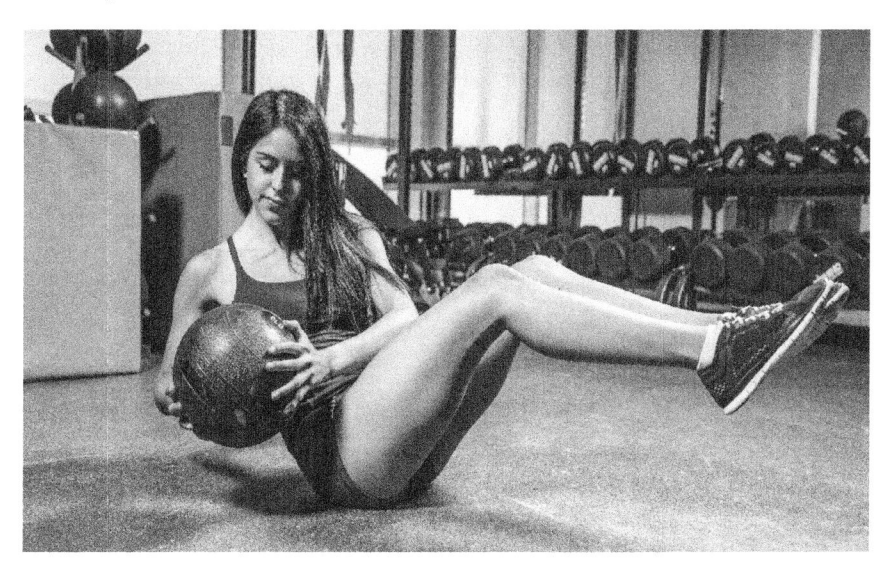

4. Alternating Toe Touches
   Lie down on your mat with your arms extended straight out to the side slightly above shoulder level. Lift your left leg and your right arm at the same time. Reach across your body to touch your left toes with your right hand. Return to the starting position and repeat on the other side. You can also complete this exercise in a standing position, either bending to touch alternate toes or alternatively lifting each leg up and touching your toes with the opposite hand.

5. Side Plank Dips
   Lie on your right side, with your elbow underneath your shoulder and your forearm perpendicular to your body, or

with your hand directly beneath your shoulder. Both legs should be extended out with either your feet staggered for more stability or stacked one on top of the other. Squeeze your glutes, engage your core and lift your hips off the floor to form a straight line from your head to your feet. Dip your hips towards the floor and then return back to a straight side plank position. Complete 10/20/30 repetitions before repeating for the same number of repetitions on your left side.

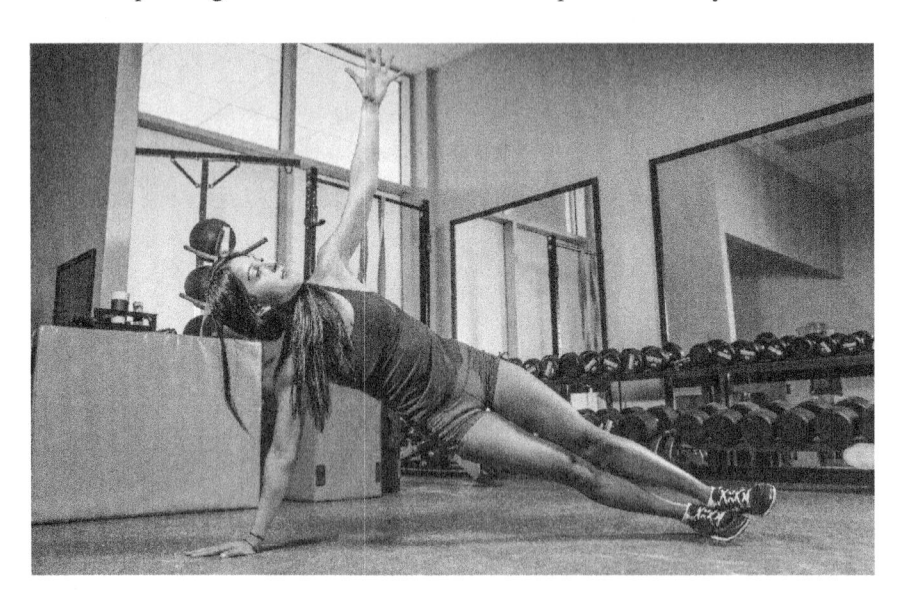

6. Plank with Knee Tucks
   Hold your preferred plank position (on your forearms or on your hands with your arms straight). Bring your right knee up towards your right elbow and flex slightly towards your right side. Return to your starting position before repeating on the other side.

7. Dead bug
   Lie on your back on the floor with your arms and legs in the air, knees bent at 90 degrees. Maintaining contact between your lower back and the floor, engage your core, then slowly

and simultaneously lower your right leg until your heel nearly touches floor and your left arm until your hand nearly touches the floor overhead. Pause, then return to the starting position before repeating on the other side.

Section 7
1. Flutter Kicks
   Lie on your back on a mat. Lift and extend your legs up to a 45-degree angle. Keep your arms straight by your sides, palms facing down. Lift your head, neck and shoulders slightly off the ground. Criss-cross your legs over one another in a scissor movement or alternatively move them up and down so that first your right leg is higher than your left and then switch so that your left is higher than your right. Flutter up and down, making sure that your lower back is pressed into the mat.

2. Sit-ups
   Lie flat on your back on a mat. Bend your knees and position your feet firmly on the mat and place your hands behind your head. Engage your core by drawing your belly button in towards your spine. Keeping your heels firmly planted on the floor, slowly lift your head and torso off the floor. Lengthen your spine to sit up tall. Return to your starting position and repeat.

3. Extension to Cannonball
   Get into a cannonball-type shape on your back, hugging your knees into your chest. Engage your core and, pressing your lower back into the mat, extend your legs and arms straight outwards, without your hands and feet touching the floor. Return to the starting position and repeat.

4. V-Ups
   Sit on your mat, embracing your knees to your chest. Engage your core and stretch out your arms and legs into a V shape.

Return to the starting position and repeat. In order to increase difficulty, you can start from a lying position and, in one movement, lift your torso and legs up into the V position. Return to the starting position and repeat.

5. Crunches

    Lie on your back. Plant your feet on the floor, hip-width apart, knees bent. Place your hands flat across your chest or behind your head. Engage your core and inhale. Exhale and lift your upper body, keeping your head and neck relaxed. Inhale and return to the starting position before repeating.

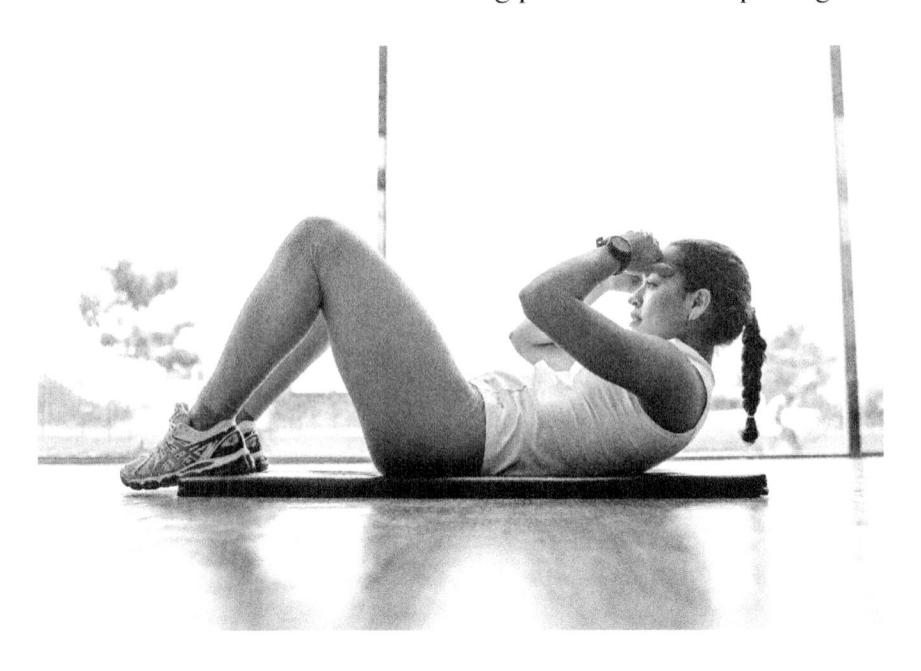

6. Reach Crunches

    Lie on your back with your legs at a 90-degree angle off the floor with your toes pointed towards the ceiling. Engage your core and inhale. Exhale and lift your upper body, stretching your hands up towards your toes. Inhale and return to the starting position before repeating.

7. Leg Lifts
   Lie on your back with your legs off the floor and pointing to the ceiling. Your arms are at your sides with the palms facing down. Engage your core and lift your lower back off the floor as your legs reach up, stretching towards the ceiling. Return to the starting position and repeat.

Now that we have explored when, why and what to eat and how to upgrade our metabolism, it's time to put all four pillars of The BODYBLISS Protocol together.

Chapter Five – THE PROTOCOL

We have now covered the four pillars of *The BODYBLISS Protocol*, namely timing, mindset, nutrition and metabolism. It's now time to put them all together into one easy plan. We're going to recap on all the main factors of each separate pillar and create one easy-to-follow protocol that is simple to apply, does not require much commitment, but delivers disproportionate, tangible, life-enhancing results.

Step One: TIMING
Our first step towards better health and easier weight management starts with timing. Optimum health is a question of balance and a respect for the body's cycles, in particular for its circadian rhythm, which divides many processes in the body between an active daylight mode and a regenerative night-time mode.

We learnt that digestion is best reserved for the daytime mode because metabolism of food becomes less efficient as evening draws on and, if the body is forced to digest food late in the evening, this will disrupt repair cycles. Eating late in the evening, as well as other stimulatory activities like watching television or working on screens, can delay the release of melatonin and HGH, which aid regenerative sleep and repair processes.

Sleep is a vital daily phase of rest and regeneration to repair the wear and tear on the body simply from being alive, active and breathing. A good night's sleep is an essential component for optimum health and easy weight management. Sleep deprivation has been proven to have a detrimental effect on weight; it creates hormonal imbalances that drive over-eating and weight gain.

> A good night's sleep is an essential component for optimum health and easy weight management.

Our protocol recommends keeping all eating within a maximum window of twelve hours and completing this 12-hour timeslot a few hours before bedtime so as not to interfere with the body's preparation for sleep. Just this one tool of keeping all eating within a 12-hour window has been shown to mitigate dietary excesses, reinforce the efficiencies inherent in the circadian rhythm and render weight management effortless.

In order to optimise the health and weight management benefits of respecting your circadian rhythm, the following ten key steps in the timing protocol are highly recommended:

1. Get exposure to bright light in the morning, preferably sunlight;
2. Keep all eating within a maximum time window of 12 hours;
3. For increased weight loss, reduce your time window for all eating down to 10 or 8 hours (so, for an 8-hour timeslot, if you have breakfast at 10am, you will finish all eating for the day by 6pm. This timeslot can be shifted earlier or later according to your individual convenience);
4. Get into the habit of drinking 1-2 glasses of water before a meal;

5. Keep the frequency of meals to a maximum of 3 a day (remember that every time you eat, you are triggering the release of insulin, which inhibits fat loss, so it is preferable to eat 2 to 3 satisfying, preferably low-glycaemic meals rather than 5 to 6 snacks);
6. Eat your largest meal at lunchtime when the body's digestion and metabolism of food is at its most efficient. Make dinner the lightest meal of the day (or skip altogether if you are narrowing your feeding window to 8 hours) as the body is at its most insulin inefficient in the evening;
7. Complete all meals by 8pm at the latest;
8. Dim lighting in the evenings and reduce screen time to an absolute minimum;
9. Balance daily stress with stress-relieving activities, such as a relaxing chat with positive friends, meditation, a yoga session, a warm bath, a walk in nature, a feel-good film, a massage or just a break from activity to let your thoughts drift;
10. Try to keep to a regular bedtime that allows for 8 hours sleep.

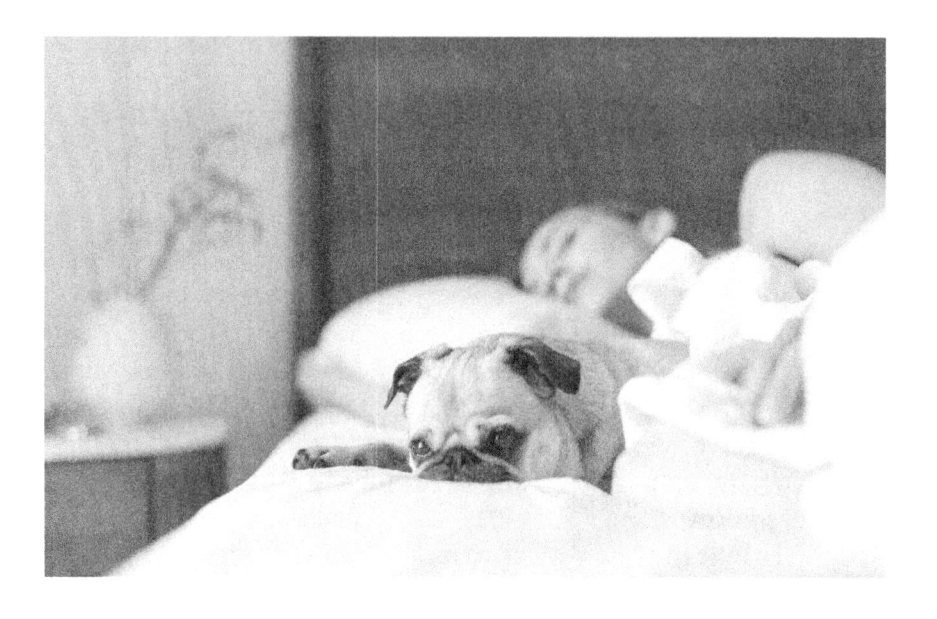

Therefore, based on the above recommendations, an ideal daily schedule might look like the following:

7.30 - 8am	Wake up Exercise routine (preferably outdoors in the sunlight)
9 - 9.15am	Breakfast Work
12.30 - 1pm	Lunch Work
5.30 - 6pm	Dinner A walk in nature A chat with friends
8 - 8.30pm	Switch off all screens and Wi-Fi for the evening Read a book, take a warm bath, relax

10.30 - 11pm Bedtime

As with all recommendations in this book, exceptions will arise, but as long as they are kept as exceptions and don't become your normality, the regular habit of respecting a 12-hour maximum window for all eating will ensure that you are doing your best to support the body's health, by respecting its cycles and its need for balance, while priming its in-built weight management function.

Step Two: MINDSET
Our second step towards better health and easier weight management is to understand why we eat. The body requires food for survival and a series of physiological cues ensure that we feel the urge to eat. However, these physiological cues can sometimes be tipped off balance and they can also very often be obscured by psychological cues. Managing and balancing our mindset provides the key to

disempowering the physiological and psychological cues that can throw our eating and weight management off balance.

The mindset protocol encompasses 4 main goals: stress relief, mindfulness (to bring greater awareness to our thoughts, emotions and actions), visualisation (a meditative exercise to improve and reprogram self-image and consequently the body's blueprint) and focus (a shift away from the attention monopoly of weight towards real purpose). The following activities help to rebalance the physiological and psychological cues that destabilise healthy eating:

1. Incorporate a few enjoyable, stress-relieving activities into your day. These offset all the stress of our days and allow us to feel good. Examples include a yoga session, meditation, taking a walk in nature, catching up with friends for some good belly laughs, watching a fun film, reading a good book, taking a warm, relaxing bath or having a massage. The key is to choose those activities that have a maximum stress-relieving effect for you.

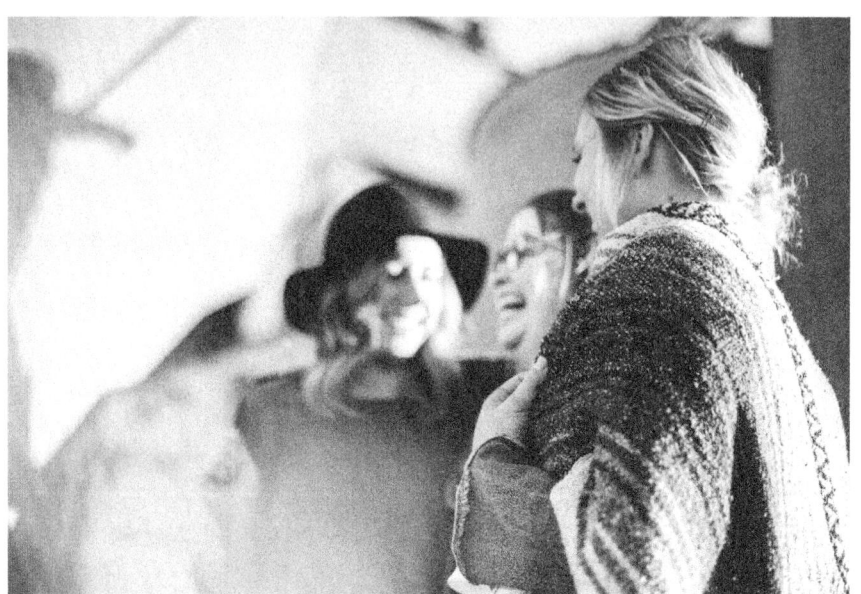

2. When you eat, do not engage in any other activity. Focus solely on what you are eating; savour the colours, the texture, the smell and the flavours. Practice gratitude and appreciation for the food you eat and for the nourishment it provides.
3. Express complete acceptance, appreciation and gratitude for your body, for all the ways in which it facilitates and supports your experience of life.
4. Accept any ways in which you may not have made the best choices for yourself. Each breath is a new opportunity to make a better choice. Forgive yourself and let any self-critical thoughts drift off.
5. Shift your inner dialogue from inner critic to inner friend or mentor. Be kind and compassionate with yourself as you would be to your dearest friend. Encourage and nurture yourself.
6. Visualise yourself feeling happy and confident in your skin. Imagine yourself walking on a beach, feel the warmth of the sun on your skin, the freshness of the water on your feet, a light breeze caressing your skin. Notice how comfortable and relaxed you feel. Imagine the shape of your body, how great your body feels as you move. This is you.
7. Find a photo of yourself at a time when your weight was your healthiest, when you were fit and strong, happy and confident. Display this photo somewhere you will see it and look at it every day, perhaps on your fridge door. Relive how you felt in this body. This is you.
8. Engage in a hobby or activity that you really love so much that it makes you sometimes lose track of time.
9. Listen to music you love every day, dance and sing.
10. Develop your unique gifts or talents with daily practice and focus.
11. Think of ways in which you could bring more joy to yourself and others.
12. Think of ways in which you could be of service to your family, your community and to the world.

By making the above activities an integral and enjoyable part of our day, we will gain mastery over the area of weight management that previously may have seemed completely out of our control. The knock-on positive effect on other parts of life that suffered as a result of deregulated eating or an unhealthy obsession with weight is a welcome side effect.

Step Three: NUTRITION
By keeping all eating within an 8- to 12-hour window and containing all eating within 2 to 3 meals, insulin levels are regularly cleared and we are activating shifts from glucose to fat metabolism on a daily basis. This timing protocol also mitigates the deleterious effects of any diet failings. However, having also learnt how to balance the physiological and psychological aspects of appetite, we are now more inclined to make the healthiest, most nutritious dietary choices to best care for our bodies.

The following dietary recommendations will remove the usual misery and sense of deprivation that most of us associate with going on a diet and will make attaining and maintaining ideal weight easy and enjoyable.

1. Cook from scratch using fresh, local produce where possible. Each of us needs to find a number of healthy, go-to meals that work according to our individual tastes and interest in cooking. Check out the recipes in Chapter Three as a guide; let them inspire you to create your own nutritious meals that are easy to make and delicious to eat.
2. Make sure that your diet contains sufficient protein. Around 0.8g of protein per kilogram of weight should be sufficient unless you are training beyond the parameters of this protocol. If you struggle to integrate sufficient protein from your diet, try adding a protein shake.
3. Protein inhibits ghrelin and NPY (hunger signals) and stimulates CCK, PYY and GLP-1 (satiety signals) more than fat or carbohydrates. It also consumes more energy to digest

and slows down the absorption of glucose into the bloodstream. So, make sure every meal contains a good source of protein.
4. Fat increases CCK levels, which increase satiety. Fat is also an essential nutrient, so it is important to integrate a good source of fat into every meal.
5. Dilute a tablespoon of apple cider vinegar in a glass of water and drink before meals.
6. Ensure your diet has sufficient fibre by eating plenty of vegetables, whole grains and fruit. Fibre slows down the absorption of glucose into the bloodstream; it, therefore, helps prevent insulin resistance. Fibre increases levels of short-chain fatty acids in the gut, which induce satiety, improve insulin sensitivity, cholesterol levels, metabolic health and gut health.
7. The following nutrients facilitate weight management. Integrate them through your diet or in a high-quality supplement:
    - ✓ Serum vitamin D levels are inversely related to BMI and body fat mass. Vitamin D inhibits lipogenesis and fat storage. It regulates serotonin synthesis and increases testosterone levels, both of which aid weight management. Ghrelin levels are higher in people with a vitamin D deficiency. Make sure you have sufficient vitamin D by getting around 15 minutes exposure to sunlight every day and eating fatty fish, like mackerel or salmon.
    - ✓ Iodine is critical for healthy thyroid function, metabolism and thermogenesis. It also helps reverse insulin resistance.
    - ✓ Chromium enhances the action of insulin, thus aiding the body to maintain normal blood glucose levels.
    - ✓ Niacin (vitamin B3) reduces LDL cholesterol, triglyceride and lipoprotein levels, while increasing HDL cholesterol levels. It plays a vital role in cellular metabolism, mitochondrial function and DNA repair.

- ✓ Magnesium is essential in the production and transfer of energy. It is useful in cases of fatigue, improving exercise performance and counteracting insomnia. It activates enzymes essential for protein and carbohydrate metabolism and it is required for the synthesis and function of DNA. It also helps counteract insulin resistance.
- ✓ L-carnitine, or acetyl-l-carnitine, is crucial for the transportation of fatty acids into the mitochondria, as well as efficient energy production. By inducing fatty acid oxidation, l-carnitine can be a useful aid to weight loss. It also improves insulin sensitivity.
- ✓ Eat foods high in melatonin or tryptophan (that can be converted into serotonin and melatonin), such as eggs, fish, poultry, dairy foods, nuts, seeds, bananas, pineapples, oranges and cherries;
- ✓ Keep serotonin levels high through exposure to sunlight, exercise, positive social interaction and by supplementing with 5-HTP, a serotonin precursor, which has been found to reduce appetite and food cravings.
- ✓ Adiponectin breaks down fat reserves. The following botanicals promote the action of adiponectin: curcumin in turmeric, capsaicin in chillis and cayenne pepper, gingerol in ginger and catechins in green tea. Try to integrate these into your daily diet.
- ✓ Vitamin C is essential for the production of oxytocin, the feel-good hormone that is so powerful for counterbalancing stress. Good sources of vitamin C include citrus fruits, berries, broccoli, peas and cauliflower.
- ✓ Isolated amino acids, such as arginine, glutamine and lysine, have been found to enhance the release of human growth hormone from the pituitary gland thus supporting lean body mass, facilitating weight management and improving recovery.

- ✓ Copper is an endogenous regulator of lipolysis. Low levels of copper may reduce thyroid function and BMR, as well as increase cholesterol levels, fatigue and reduce nerve conductivity.
- ✓ Coenzyme Q10 plays an important role in the generation of energy in cell mitochondria. Endogenous levels have been seen to diminish with age. It improves exercise performance, insulin resistance, antioxidant protection, it regulates blood glucose levels and has cardioprotective properties.

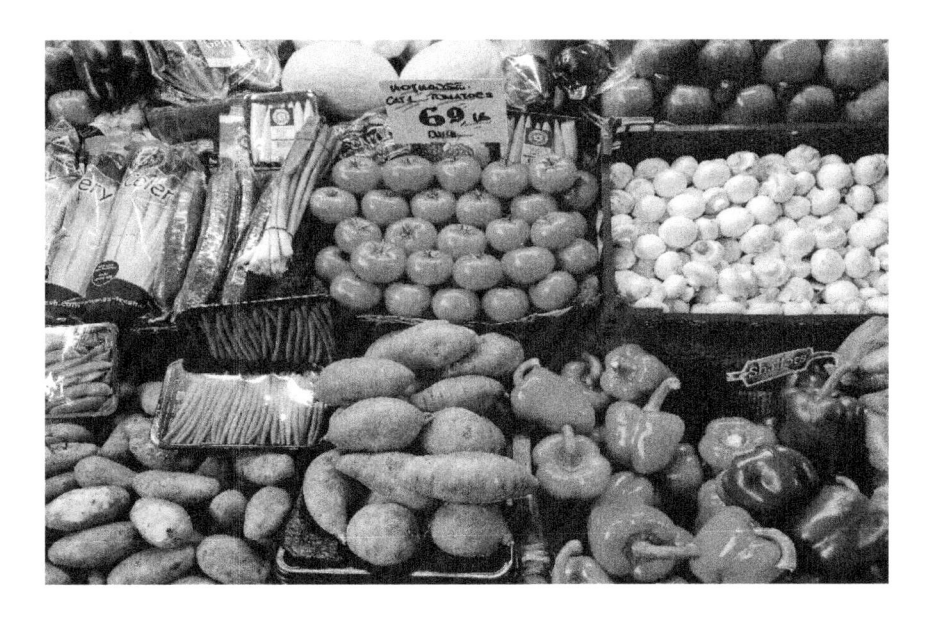

- ✓ Curcumin is well known for its anti-inflammatory properties. Some studies have highlighted the key role of inflammation in obesity as both a driver and a result. Inflammation interferes with hypothalamic signalling. Curcumin boosts brain function, serotonin and dopamine levels, endogenous antioxidant action and also has cardioprotective properties.

- ✓ Some studies have found that the high-fibre Irvingia Gabonensis seed, also known as African Mango, reduces blood glucose levels, total cholesterol and triglycerides while increasing HDL cholesterol. It is thus purported to improve insulin resistance, type 2 diabetes and facilitates weight management.
- ✓ Green tea contains caffeine, which activates some lipolysis and is purported to improve exercise performance. However, it is its high catechin content that distinguishes this nutrient, in particular epigallocatechin gallate (EPCG), which boosts antioxidant action and metabolism, as well as improving insulin sensitivity and glucose tolerance.
- ✓ Resveratrol, a phytochemical found in grapes and berries, has antioxidant, neuroprotective, cardioprotective, hepatoprotective and anti-inflammatory properties. It improves insulin sensitivity, cholesterol levels and metabolism.

All of the above nutrients can be found in the high-quality supplements MAGNESSENCE® and BODYBISS® from FIREBIRD®.

Step Four: METABOLISM
If you are currently doing no exercise, it is vital for your general health and successful weight management to start integrating some enjoyable movement into your day. Start with an easy walk. Go somewhere beautiful in nature. Making the exercise experience an enjoyable part of your day that you look forward to rather than dread having to do, is vital in order to consistently integrate it into your routine.

The following steps will contribute to strengthening your BMR, making exercise an enjoyable addition to your daily routine, developing strength and agility, giving you greater body confidence and enhancing your quality of life.

1. Introduce some exposure to the cold into your daily routine, whether it's just a cold blast under the shower, a reduction of a few degrees on the thermostat or a cold dip in the sea or bath.
2. Integrate more movement into your daily life, whether it's a walk after dinner, a pledge to use the stairs over the lift or playing tag with the kids, whatever gets you more active provides health benefits in terms of improved mood, higher self-esteem and easier weight management. Be conscious of how you engage your muscles as you move; feel your abdominal muscles, your glutes and your leg muscles contract as you walk, for example.
3. Commit to a regular exercise routine that includes aerobic, anaerobic and flexibility exercises. The aim is to have a daily practice (ideally five times a week or more) structured as below with a warm up, a sustained workout and a cool down with stretching:

Warm Up
Rotate joints (ankles, knees, pelvis, torso, arms, wrists and neck)
Marching and jogging on the spot

Workout
Aerobic exercise (e.g. walking, swimming, cycling, dancing)
High-intensity interval training (HIIT)

Stretching
Slow march on the spot or walk
Stretching

The above routine combines aerobic with anaerobic exercise along with flexibility exercises. It can be adapted according to your fitness level. An example of a beginner's routine would be a warm-up involving rotating the joints, followed by a 15- to 20-minute walk, some lunges, crunches and tricep dips, followed by some gentle stretches.

A more advanced version would involve a warm-up, rotating the joints and jogging on the spot, followed by a 20-minute run and 3 circuits of the HIIT exercises listed below, with 15 minutes of stretching or yoga to finish.

HIIT Exercises
In order to compose a workout, choose one exercise per day from each section. Start with 10 repetitions and build up to 30 or more depending on the exercise. As your fitness level improves, repeat the sequence of seven exercises twice or more times. You can also use the tabata method of completing the maximum number of repetitions in 20 or 30 seconds, followed by a 10- to 15-second break before continuing to the next exercise.

In the space of a week, try to complete all 7 exercises from each section, or at least 5, as each section targets a different set of muscles and each exercise in each section engages the targeted muscles in a different way. So, you could follow the sequence suggested taking the number one exercise from each section to make up your Monday workout (see below), take the number two exercise from each section for your Tuesday workout and so on, so that, in the space of a week, you will complete all seven exercises from each section.

Example of your Monday workout:
1. Plank Jack
2. Tricep Dips
3. Squats
4. Jumping Jacks
5. Glute Bridge
6. Elbow to Knee Crunches
7. Flutter Kicks

Sections 1 and 2 are for upper body strength, sections 3, 4 and 5 are to tone and develop the leg and glute muscles, and sections 6 and 7 are for torso strength, including developing those abdominal muscles for a much-desired six-pack.

Upper Body
Section 1
1. Plank Jacks (jump legs out to side and back)
2. Plank to Downward Dog
3. Lateral plank walk
4. Plank with shoulder taps
5. Plank to Push up
6. Plank with Arm extensions
7. Straight Plank

Section 2
1. Tricep Dips in crab position or off a chair
2. Bicep curls with weights
3. Push ups
4. Punch Ball on both sides
5. Arm Rotations with weights (arms outstretched)
6. Superman
7. Arm Lifts

Legs and Glutes
Section 3
1. Squats
2. Lunges
3. Reverse Lunges
4. Side lunges
5. 30 Plies with 30 pulses
6. Forward leg lifts
7. Backward Leg lifts

Section 4
1. Jumping Jacks
2. Karate kicks
3. Squat kicks
4. Squat jumps (touch floor and up)
5. Burpee squats

    6. Speed Skater
    7. Mountain Climber

Section 5
1. Glute bridge
2. Side Leg Lifts
3. Inner Thigh Lifts
4. Donkey kicks
5. Wide-leg glute bridge
6. Side donkey kicks
7. Seated to glute bridge

Abs
Section 6
1. Elbow to knee crunches
2. Russian twist
3. Heel taps
4. Alternating toe touches
5. Side plank dips
6. Plank with knee tucks
7. Dead bug

Section 7
1. Flutter Kicks
2. Sit-ups
3. Extension to Cannonball
4. V-Ups
5. Crunches
6. Reach Crunches
7. Leg Lifts

The BODYBLISS Protocol Journal

As you have read through this book, much of the knowledge presented may have resonated with you as intuitively true. You may have accepted intellectually that *The BODYBLISS Protocol* is the system you have been looking for, the system that will finally make weight management so easy that you no longer have to even think about it and you can just get on with your life. In order for this to be true, we have to engage with the subconscious mind to such an extent that this system becomes an automatic habit. This is achieved by creating habitual behaviour. *The BODYBLISS Protocol Journal* is the habit-forming tool recommended to engage with your subconscious mind and turn this system into second nature for you.

It is believed that any behaviour requires between a few and several weeks of assiduous practice before it can become an ingrained habit. *The BODYBLISS Protocol Journal* gives you the framework to keep tabs on your compliance, track your progress and highlight any issues. Once a week, you will be given the opportunity to review your progress, course correct, if necessary, recalibrate your focus and plot your direction for the week ahead.

The table at the end of this chapter is a page from *The BODYBLISS Protocol Journal*, which helps track the elements involved in *The BODYBLISS Protocol* that contribute to optimal health and ideal weight.

Each day you will enter your weight at the top of the page. This is a tracking exercise that confirms your progress, your stability or provides an early warning detection point if you are starting to veer off course. Your weight can fluctuate from day to day, but a steady increase or decrease over the course of a week usually highlights a trend. The journal allows you to look back over the last week to identify the elements that may have contributed to this trend.

The TIMING box firstly asks about your sleep. Did you sleep well? This is a yes or no answer. If the answer is no, you might want to check what elements from the day before may have contributed to you not getting a good night's sleep. Did you go to bed later than usual? Did you have dinner later than usual? Were you more stressed than usual? Did you sit up watching television? How can you ensure that you will sleep better tonight?

The rest of the TIMING box entries refer to times: What time did you have breakfast? What time did you finish dinner? How many hours was your eating window (completion of dinnertime minus breakfast time, for example, 19h (7pm) – 8h (8am) = 11 hours)? What time did you switch off all screens? What time did you go to bed?

The MINDSET box requires more thought. You can use this section to plan your day and record what you achieved. So, for relaxation, list the activities you will engage in to counterbalance any stress in your day. Examples could include yoga, a walk by the sea and meditation. This list is the plan; you can then tick off what you actually did.

The mindful eating entry is an assessment of whether you ate your meals mindfully without doing some other activity at the same time. If you enter two ticks and a cross, this would mean you practised mindful eating during two meals, but combined eating with something else on the third meal.

The gratitude list allows space for you to keep note of what you are most grateful for in your life. It can be something different every day or the same, but always take a moment to fully feel your appreciation and thankfulness for every entry on your list.

Self-care and kindness refer to the ways in which you are looking after yourself. If you are someone who takes care of everyone else before you think of yourself, this section forces you to find ways each day to be kind and caring to yourself too. There may be some crossover between this and other sections of the MINDSET box, but try to really use this list to start to identify all the ways in which you could be more caring and kind towards yourself.

The visualisation entry is to check whether you completed your visualisation exercise. Take some time with this; make it a fun, enjoyable experience. The more emotional input you pour into imagining yourself at your best, the more compelled you will be to match this vision for yourself in reality.

The creativity/joy/fun entry is to check whether you are developing your sense of passion and adventure. This section is just for fun. Did you put some of your favourite music on? Did you sing and dance? Did you knit, doodle, paint, cook, write or draw just for the fun of it with no pressure to be any good? Did you explore some topic just to discover more about it? Did you make a daisy chain? Did you play with your kids? All these activities feed your soul and add to your happiness quota, which reduces the incentive salience of food.

The connection/love list ensures that you are in touch with others, people you love and care for. Did you call your parents? Did you send your best friend a message? Did you invite a friend round for dinner? How did you express your love for someone today? Cultivating connection and love is a big reason why we are all here. By prioritising this aspect of our lives and checking in with it every day, we ensure that the busyness of life is not obscuring what is really important.

The Priorities/Focus/Purpose/Service list allows us to define what, if we completed, would give us a sense of achievement and purpose. This can be something related to work, to a hobby, to your family and friends; whatever is really important for you to do today goes here. Examples might include clearing out the spare room, completing a specific work project, accompanying your daughter to her hockey match, writing a poem or calling someone about a work opportunity. These are all actions that you prioritise that move you in the direction of your purpose. Ticking these off gives you the satisfaction to record that you completed the priorities you defined for your day. You can add the outstanding actions on your list to the next day or you can re-evaluate their importance to your intention of living a life of purpose and value.

In the NUTRITION box, you will record how many times you ate and check or cross whether you included a good source of protein in your meals, whether you ate fruit and vegetables, healthy fat, fibre, whether you drank some diluted apple cider vinegar before at least one meal and whether you remembered to take your supplements. This box purposefully requires a low input from you. It intentionally shifts the focus away from exactly what you ate to whether you sufficiently nourished your body. Your focus is on building a valuable life and not on keeping track of calories.

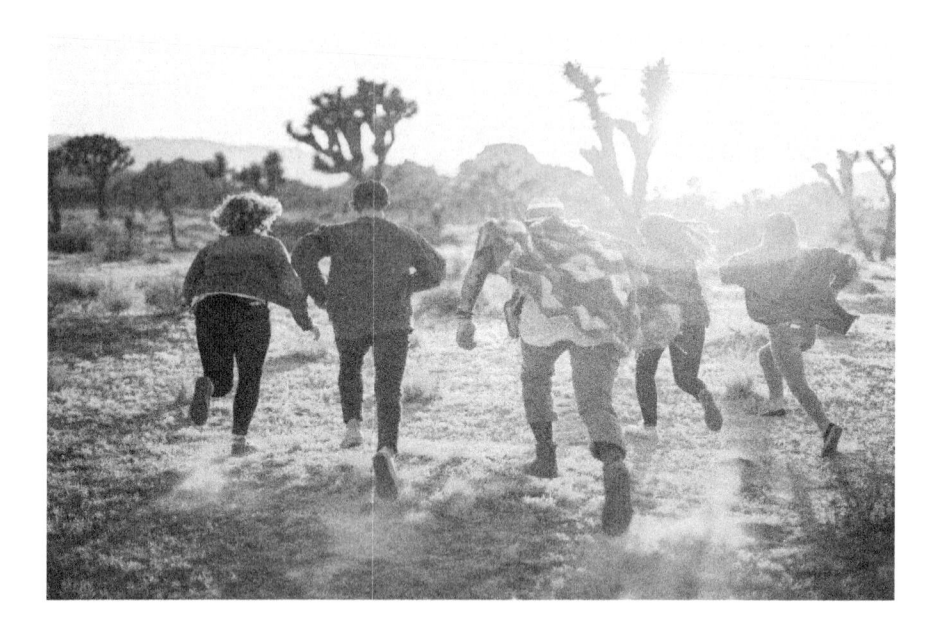

In the METABOLISM box, you can keep track of whether you are doing everything you can to support a healthy metabolism, cardiovascular health, flexibility and high energy. The first entry is a yes or no response to whether you had any cold exposure; did you give yourself a cold blast under the shower? Did you go for a swim in the sea? For the aerobic entry you might enter a 20-minute walk to work or a 45-minute dance session. For the anaerobic exercise section, seven lines are given to enter which HIIT exercises you completed, for example, you might enter 30 plank jacks, 20 tricep dips, 20 squats, 30 jumping jacks, 30 glute bridges, 40 elbow-to-knee crunches and 20 flutter kicks. The flexibility exercise entry might just include ten minutes of stretching.

Every seventh day in *The BODYBLISS Protocol Journal*, you have a chance to review your progress and study what changes you would like to make for the week ahead. *The BODYBLISS Protocol Journal* allows you to plan in advance, determine your focus for the week, align with your goals and celebrate those goals achieved.

Now that you have the tools for making weight management easy, your health and weight no longer require obsessive attention. *The BODYBLISS Protocol* has hopefully freed your focus from the all-consuming obsession of weight-watching and allowed you to rediscover what you really want your life to be about. *The BODYBLISS Protocol Journal* can really help you keep aligned with that new direction every day while moving towards ever better health and effortless weight management.

TIMING

A Good Night's Sleep YES/NO

Breakfast..........................

Dinner Completed...............

Window..........................

Digital Curfew...................

Bedtime..........................

MINDSET

Relaxation
....
....
....

Mindful Eating   YES/NO

Gratitude
....
....
....

Self-care & Kindness
....
....

Visualisation   YES/NO

Creativity/Joy/Fun
....
....

Connection/Love
....
....

Priorities/Focus/Purpose
....
....
....

Date:..................................

Weight:........................

NUTRITION

Number of Meals............

Protein	YES/NO
Fruit & vegetables	YES/NO
Healthy Fat	YES/NO
Fibre	YES/NO
Apple Cider Vinegar	YES/NO
Supplements	YES/NO

METABOLISM

Cold Exposure   YES/NO

Aerobic Exercise
- ✓ ....
- ✓ ....

Anaerobic Exercise
1. ....
2. ....
3. ....
4. ....
5. ....
6. ....
7. ....

Flexibility Exercise
- ✓ ....
- ✓ ....

Conclusion

We have followed the journey of weight management from when we eat and why we eat to the importance of what we eat. We now understand that weight management is a complex symphony orchestrated by a multitude of players that, if kept in balance, perpetuate optimal health, mental stability and easy weight management. We know that the excess expression or erroneous timing of any one player can throw the whole symphony off key and make perfect health and weight management so much more difficult to attain and maintain.

We have learnt that the interplay of hunger and satiety signals are intended to keep weight balanced, but that, quite often, whether through physiological or psychological factors, these signals can become deregulated and tip the weight balance. Certain foods cause overexpression of hunger signals while others are more effective at attenuating hunger. We have learnt that the nutritional composition of food triggers specific hormones and metabolic pathways that determine whether they are more or less conducive to weight management.

Previous dietary advice recommended 6 to 11 servings of carbohydrates a day, preferably spaced out in 6 or more meals and snacks. Low-fat options were strongly endorsed, in which fat content was usually replaced with sugar. However, while fat is satiating, sugar activates the dopamine reward system and triggers cravings. Calories were the dominant consideration and measure of balance, despite knowledge that a bottle of cola, for example, may have the same calories as a handful of nuts, but the metabolic journey in the body of each option is quite distinct.

In recent decades, we have been exposed to and consumed more and more calorie-dense, processed foods made with a combination of sugar, salt, fat and carbohydrate that are particularly efficient at triggering the reward centres of the brain and activating addictive cravings, which drive us to consume excessive quantities of these foods and confound weight management. Alternative methods of weight management have to be employed to deal with these addictive cravings that go beyond the normal parameters of diet plans, but which we have addressed in *The BODYBLISS Protocol*.

In the past, weight management has been reduced to an energy equation. Diet guidelines have mainly advocated creating an energy deficit by eating less and exercising more. However, caloric restriction, when put into practice, drives down the body's BMR, making weight loss harder and harder to achieve. These recommendations and others, such as low-fat diets, have not yielded the desired results and obesity is fast reaching epidemic levels in developed countries.

> Caloric restriction, when put into practice, drives down the body's BMR, making weight loss harder and harder to achieve.

Not only is it important to understand the physiological effects on the body of what we eat, it is also of utmost importance to understand how meal frequency compounds these effects. In Chapter One, we studied timing and learnt that weight management is easier if we respect our circadian rhythm and eat within a window of twelve hours. For weight loss, this window is best limited to 8 hours around midday. This is because our metabolism's efficiency changes throughout the day such that a doughnut eaten first thing in the morning has a lower effect on blood glucose than the same doughnut eaten later in the day, when its effect on blood glucose would be greater and therefore its potential to be stored as fat is also higher. This is because insulin resistance rises in the evening. So, ideally, if we have breakfast at 8am, for example, we need to finish eating for the day by 4pm. It is also better to have 2 or 3 meals as opposed to more frequent snacks that trigger insulin each time and reduce fat oxidation.

Through the course of this book, we have seen that a more holistic approach to weight management is required. Easy, effective weight management is the result of both lifestyle and dietary modifications that facilitate hormonal balance, stress management, emotional balance, high quality sleep, efficient metabolism and sufficient rest and repair. The body functions optimally if we respect its cycles and need for balance. In fact, practising TRF alone can mitigate the most harmful effects of an unhealthy diet. This is the reason why it is given prime position in the diagram below, which illustrates the factors required for optimum weight management.

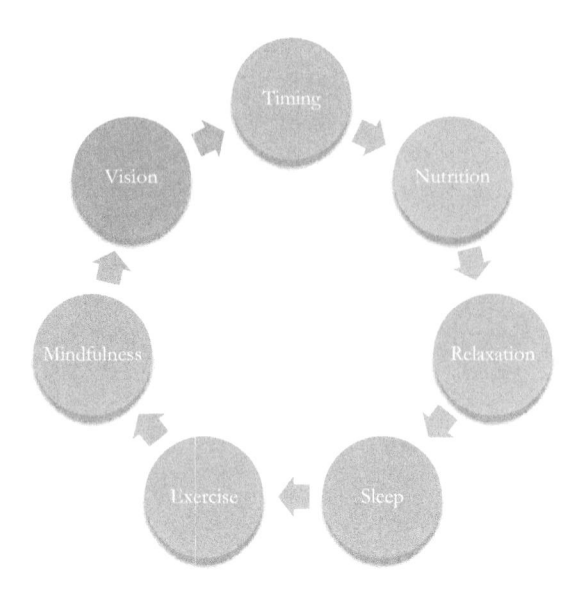

Fig. 2: Holistic Weight Management

Effective weight management must take into account the above 7 elements.
1. **Timing**: this factor recognises that the body's metabolism is more efficient in the morning and it needs a 12-hour rest period. So, for weight loss, an individual can eat 2/3 meals within an 8-hour window around noon; for weight management, an individual should try to eat no more than 3 meals a day including snacks within a 12-hour window. Late-night eating is not recommended. As long as these guidelines are respected 90% of the time, they can be broken occasionally.
2. **Nutrition**: the aim of diet is to provide optimum nutrition so that the body can maintain optimum health. This does not involve calorie counting, but instead, generally trying to find the healthiest options in any situation. It involves favouring

high quality protein, essential fats and a wide variety of fruit and vegetables.
3. **Relaxation**: chronic stress drives weight gain. Therefore, it is essential to find ways to reduce stress levels and/or find ways to balance stress by making time every day for relaxing activities. Whatever makes you personally relax, feel at ease, light and joyful, strong and comfortable, at peace and happy, is vital to wellness and effective weight management. Examples include yoga, meditation, a walk, a warm bath, watching a comedy, catching up with friends or a massage.
4. **Sleep**: this is not an optional, but instead an integral part of health and a vital key to effective weight management. Good quality sleep largely depends upon establishing a routine; a regular bedtime preceded by a couple of hours spent winding down towards sleep is ideal in order to maximise melatonin and human growth hormone release, both essential players in the repair and regenerative function of sleep. Minimising evening stress, blue-light exposure and heavy evening meals can help maximise melatonin release and ensure a good night's sleep.
5. **Exercise**: in weight loss circles, exercise was traditionally aimed at creating an energy deficit. In our paradigm, exercise is aimed at maximising cardiovascular health, muscular strength, BMR and hormonal balance. Daily burst training can be combined with some aerobic sessions (a swim, a brisk walk, a dance session) and weight training, including body-weight exercises. Stretching and posture work are also useful for flexibility and body confidence.
6. **Mindfulness**: this practice aims to bring unhealthy, subconscious habits into consciousness. It involves breathing exercises, slowing down, focusing one's attention on present actions. It helps us become aware of the thoughts and feelings that are driving unhealthy habits, allowing time and space to observe and accept them. Mindful eating involves not combining eating with other activities, such as working on a computer, scrolling through social media, using a

smartphone, reading or watching television. Mindful eating involves savouring the food that is being eaten, chewing well and being conscious of signals of satiety and fullness.
7. **Vision**: our habits are driven by the vision we have of ourselves. Our vision acts as a blueprint determining which actions are coherent with that vision and which actions are not. If we envision ourselves as healthy, active, lithe, agile, strong and vibrant, we are more likely to act accordingly, choosing healthy foods to eat, exercising daily, integrating more activity and time outdoors into our day. It will influence the way we dress and hold ourselves, how well we take care of ourselves and how well we interact with others.

The above system seeks to ensure optimum nutrition and metabolic health. It also aims to improve mental health and wellbeing. It can take us from a feeling of hopelessness over weight back to a position of balance and easy weight management. The major strength of this system is its ease of practice; there are no calories to count, no rigid menus to stick to, no lists of forbidden foods, no gruelling training schedules. It is easier to set a feeding window of 8-12 hours and stick to it rather than placing limits on food choices. The system requires the integration of a sleep routine, some daily exercise, daily relaxation, limiting food intake to 2/3 meals with a gradual tendency towards selecting healthier, more nutritious choices, a mindfulness practice and a new vision of a healthy self. All of these tools are pleasurable, providing the reward aspects that were previously sought through food intake. They guarantee better health and easy, effective weight management.

A realignment of focus on new goals is also a crucial aim of *The BODYBLISS Protocol*. Where weight has become an issue in life, it tends to monopolise our focus and become a determining factor of our behaviour in everyday life. No one was born with the life purpose of losing weight and yet, for so many, weight and the need to lose weight, becomes the main life focus. This book's principal aim is to free us all from the tyranny of weight, to render weight management so easy and effortless that we can refocus our attention on more inspiring goals. We were all born to be and do something more significant than manage our weight. If you make this protocol an integral part of your life, you will not only attain and maintain your ideal weight effortlessly, but you will also free yourself from all thoughts regarding weight so that you can start living a more vibrant, purposeful life, guided by a stronger awareness, a sharper focus and a tighter connection with your real priorities.

This is my wish for you all. I would love to hear how you get on and, in the meantime, enjoy the journey!

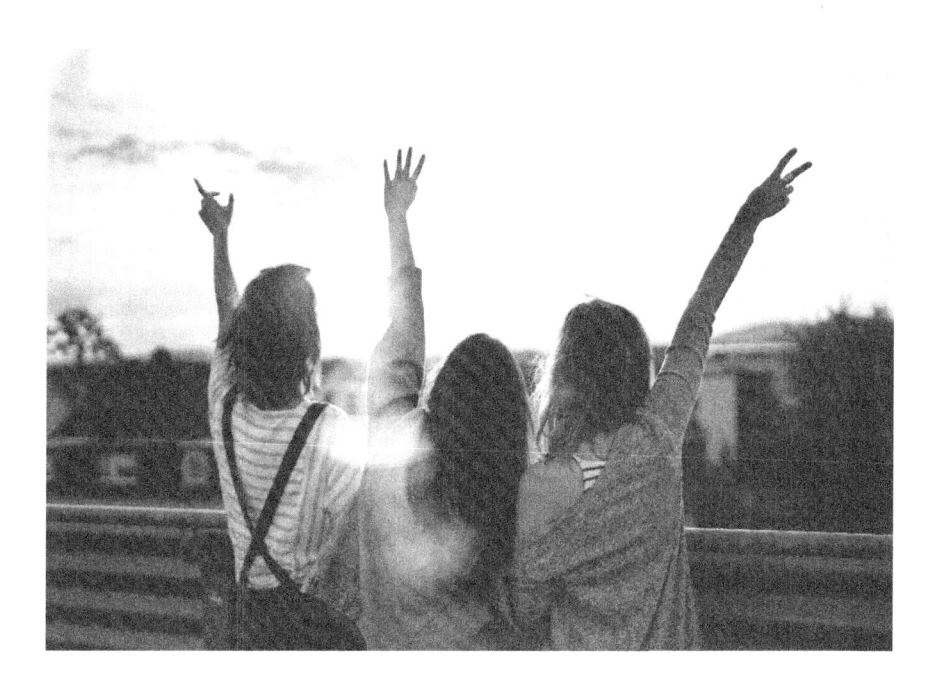

References

Introduction

1. Wing RR, Phelan S. Long-term weight loss maintenance. Am J Clin Nutr 2005; 82 (suppl):222S–5S.
2. Wing RR, Hill JO. Successful weight loss maintenance. Annu Rev Nutr 2001;21:323–41.
3. Flegal KM, Carroll MD, Ogden CL, Johnson CL 2002 Prevalence and trends in obesity among US adults, 1999–2000. JAMA 288:1723–1727
4. Bourne J 2001 Tackling obesity in England. 1–72. 7-2-2001. London: National Audit Office
5. Leonard WR. Food for thought: Dietary change was a driving force in human evolution. Sci. Am. 2002; 287(6):106–115.
6. Leonard WR, Robertson ML. Evolutionary perspectives on human nutrition: The influence of brain and body size on diet and metabolism. Am J Hum Biol. 1994; 6:77–88.
8. Crawford MA. The role of dietary fatty acids in biology: Their place in the evolution of the human brain. Nutr Rev. 1992;50:3–11.
10. Jonathan C. K. Wells. The evolution of human adiposity and obesity: where did it all go wrong? Disease Models & Mechanisms 2012. 5: 595-607;
11. Frisancho AR. Reduced rate of fat oxidation: A metabolic pathway to obesity in the developing nations. Am J Hum Biol. 2003; 15:35–52.
12. Friedman JM. A war on obesity, not the obese. Science. 2003; 299(5608):856-8.
13. Jean Ferrières. The French paradox: lessons for other countries. Heart. 2004 Jan; 90(1): 107–111.
14. Criqui MH, Ringel BL. Does diet or alcohol explain the French paradox? Lancet. 1994 Dec 24-31;344(8939-8940):1719-23.
15. Jose Manuel Lerma-Cabrera, Francisca Carvajal and Patricia Lopez-Legarrea. Food addiction as a new piece of the obesity framework. Nutrition Journal 2016. 15:5.

Chapter One – Timing

1. Vitaterna MH, Takahashi JS, Turek FW. Overview of circadian rhythms. Alcohol Research & Health 2001. 25 (2): 85–93.
2. Bass J. Circadian topology of metabolism. Nature 2012. 491 (7424): 348–56.
3. Dijk DJ, von Schantz M. Timing and consolidation of human sleep, wakefulness, and performance by a symphony of oscillators. Journal of Biological Rhythms 2005. 20 (4): 279–90.

4. Sharma VK. Adaptive significance of circadian clocks. Chronobiology International 2003. 20 (6): 901–19.
5. Kyriacou CP. Physiology. Unravelling traveling. Science 2009. 325 (5948): 1629–30.
6. J Sajan, TA Cinu, AJ Chacko, J Litty and T Jaseeda. Chronotherapeutics and Chronotherapeutic Drug Delivery Systems. Tropical Journal of Pharmaceutical Research, 2009. 8 (5): 467-475.
7. Wirz-Justice A, Benedetti F, Berger M, Lam RW, Martiny K, Terman M, Wu JC. Chronotherapeutics (light and wake therapy) in affective disorders. Psychol Med. 2005. 35(7):939-44.
8. Duffy JF, Wright KP. Entrainment of the human circadian system by light. Journal of Biological Rhythms 2005. 20 (4): 326–38.
9. Benloucif S, Guico MJ, Reid KJ, Wolfe LF, L'Hermite M, Zee PC. Stability of melatonin and temperature as circadian phase markers and their relation to sleep times in humans. Journal of Biological Rhythms 2005. 20 (2): 178–88.
10. Welsh DK, Takahashi JS, Kay SA. Suprachiasmatic nucleus: cell autonomy and network properties. Annual Review of Physiology 2010. 72: 551–77.
11. Valenzuela FJ, Vera J, Venegas C, Muñoz S, Oyarce S, Muñoz K, Lagunas C. Evidences of Polymorphism Associated with Circadian System and Risk of Pathologies: A Review of the Literature. Int J Endocrinol. 2016;2016:2746909.
12. Scott EM, Carter AM, Grant PJ. Association between polymorphisms in the Clock gene, obesity and the metabolic syndrome in man. International Journal of Obesity 2008. 32 (4): 658–62.
13. Nelson RJ, Chbeir S. Dark matters: effects of light at night on metabolism. Proc Nutr Soc. 2018 May 11:1-7.
14. Fonken LK, Aubrecht TG, Meléndez-Fernández OH, Weil ZM, Nelson RJ. Dim light at night disrupts molecular circadian rhythms and increases body weight. J Biol Rhythms. 2013 Aug;28(4):262-71.
15. Perreau-Lenz S, Pévet P, Buijs RM, Kalsbeek A. The biological clock: the bodyguard of temporal homeostasis. Chronobiol Int. 2004. 21(1):1-25.
16. Perreau-Lenz S, Kalsbeek A, Garidou ML, et al. Suprachiasmatic control of melatonin synthesis in rats: inhibitory and stimulatory mechanisms. Eur J Neurosci 2003. 17(2):221–228.
17. Pevet P, Challet E. Melatonin: both master clock output and internal time-giver in the circadian clocks network. J Physiol Paris. 2011 Dec;105(4-6):170-82.
18. Yoshizaki T, Midorikawa T, Hasegawa K, Mitani T, Komatsu T, Togo F. Associations between diurnal 24-hour rhythm in ambulatory heart rate variability and the timing and amount of meals during the day shift in rotating shift workers. PLoS One. 2014 Sep 11;9(9):e106643.

19. Fonken LK, Nelson RJ. The effects of light at night on circadian clocks and metabolism. Endocr Rev. 2014 Aug;35(4):648-70.
20. Mendoza J, Graff C, Dardente H, Pevet P, Challet E. Feeding cues alter clock gene oscillations and photic responses in the suprachiasmatic nuclei of mice exposed to a light/dark cycle. J Neurosci. 2005. 25(6):1514-22.
21. Challet E. Keeping circadian time with hormones. Diabetes Obes Metab. 2015 Sep;17 Suppl 1:76-83.
22. Mistlberger RE, Antle MC. Entrainment of circadian clocks in mammals by arousal and food. Essays Biochem. 2011 Jun 30;49(1):119-36.
23. Hardeland R. Antioxidative protection by melatonin: multiplicity of mechanisms from radical detoxification to radical avoidance. Endocrine 2005. 27 (2): 119–30.
24. Reiter RJ, Acuña-Castroviejo D, Tan DX, Burkhardt S. Free radical-mediated molecular damage. Mechanisms for the protective actions of melatonin in the central nervous system. Ann. N. Y. Acad. Sci 2001. 939: 200–15.
25. Tan DX, Manchester LC, Terron MP, Flores LJ, Reiter RJ. One molecule, many derivatives: a never-ending interaction of melatonin with reactive oxygen and nitrogen species? J. Pineal Res 2007. 42 (1): 28–42.
26. Sae-Teaw M, Johns J, Johns NP, Subongkot S. Serum melatonin levels and antioxidant capacities after consumption of pineapple, orange, or banana by healthy male volunteers. J. Pineal Res 2012. 55 (1): 58–64.
27. Carrillo-Vico A, Guerrero JM, Lardone PJ, Reiter RJ. A review of the multiple actions of melatonin on the immune system. Endocrine 2005. 27 (2): 189–200.
28. Mills E, Wu P, Seely D, Guyatt G. Melatonin in the treatment of cancer: a systematic review of randomized controlled trials and meta-analysis. J. Pineal Res 2005. 39 (4): 360–66.
29. Feychting Maria; OsterLund, Bill; Ahlbom, Anders. Reduced Cancer Incidence among the Blind. Epidemiology: September 1998.
30. Kayumov L, Casper RF, Hawa RJ, Perelman B, Chung SA, Sokalsky S, Shapiro CM. Blocking low-wavelength light prevents nocturnal melatonin suppression with no adverse effect on performance during simulated shift work. J. Clin. Endocrinol. Metab 2005. 90 (5): 2755–61.
31. Puchalski SS, Green JN, Rasmussen DD. Melatonin effect on rat body weight regulation in response to high-fat diet at middle age. Endocrine 2003. 21:163–7.
32. Wolden-Hanson T, Mitton DR, Mccants RL, Yellon SM, Wilkinson CW, Matsumoto AM, et al. Daily melatonin administration to middle-aged male rats suppresses body weight, intraabdominal adiposity, and plasma leptin and insulin independent of food intake and total body fat. Endocrinology 2000. 141:487–97.

33. Cipolla-Neto J, Amaral FG, Afeche SC, Tan DX, Reiter RJ. Melatonin, energy metabolism, and obesity: a review. J Pineal Res 2014. 56:371–81.
34. Daniella Buonfiglio, Rafaela Parthimos, Rosana Dantas, Raysa Cerqueira Silva, Guilherme Gomes, Jéssica Andrade-Silva, Angela Ramos-Lobo, Fernanda Gaspar Amaral, Raphael Matos, José Sinésio Jr., Lívia Clemente Motta-Teixeira, José Donato Jr., Russel J. Reiter and José Cipolla-Neto. Melatonin Absence Leads to Long-Term Leptin Resistance and Overweight in Rats. Front. Endocrinol. 2018.
35. Kim KR, Nam SY, Song YD, Lim SK, Lee HC, Huh KB. Low-dose growth hormone treatment with diet restriction accelerates body fat loss, exerts anabolic effect and improves growth hormone secretory dysfunction in obese adults. Horm Res. 1999. 51(2):78-84.
36. Cermakian N, Boivin DB. The regulation of central and peripheral circadian clocks in humans. Obes Rev. 2009. 10 Suppl 2:25-36.
37. Skene DJ, Arendt J. Human circadian rhythms: physiological and therapeutic relevance of light and melatonin. Ann Clin Biochem. 2006. 43(Pt 5):344-53.
38. Li Y, van den Pol AN. Direct and indirect inhibition by catecholamines of hypocretin/orexin neurons. The Journal of Neuroscience 2005. 25 (1): 173–83.
39. Sellayah D, Bharaj P, Sikder D. Orexin is required for brown adipose tissue development, differentiation, and function. Cell Metabolism 2011. 14 (4): 478–90.
40. Chemelli RM, Willie JT, Sinton CM, Elmquist JK, Scammell T, Lee C, Richardson JA, Williams SC, Xiong Y, Kisanuki Y, Fitch TE, Nakazato M, Hammer RE, Saper CB, Yanagisawa M. Narcolepsy in orexin knockout mice: molecular genetics of sleep regulation. Cell. 1999. 98(4):437-51.
41. Wei Zhang, Jinko Sunanaga, Yoshiko Takahashi, Taketsugu Mori, Takeshi Sakurai, Yuichi Kanmura, Tomoyuki Kuwaki. Orexin neurons are indispensable for stress-induced thermogenesis in mice. The Journal of Physiology 2010. Vol. 588, I21, 4117-4129.
42. Tsuneki H, Wada T, Sasaoka T. Role of orexin in the regulation of glucose homeostasis. Acta Physiologica 2010. 198 (3): 335–48.
43. Raffaella Spinazzi, Paola G. Andreis, Gian Paolo Rossi and Gastone G. Nussdorfer. Orexins in the Regulation of the Hypothalamic-Pituitary-Adrenal Axis. Pharmacological Reviews 2006. 58 (1) 46-57
44. Fabio García-Garcíam Enrique Juárez-Aguilar, Juan Santiago-García, Daniel P.Cardinali. Ghrelin and its interactions with growth hormone, leptin and orexins: Implications for the sleep–wake cycle and metabolism. Sleep Medicine Reviews 2014. Vol. 18, I1, 89-97.
45. Christopher M. Jung, Sat Bir S. Khalsa, Frank A. J. L. Scheer, Christian Cajochen, Steven W. Lockley, Charles A. Czeisler, and Kenneth P.

Wright, Jr. Acute Effects of Bright Light Exposure on Cortisol Levels. J Biol Rhythms. 2010. 25(3): 208–216.
46. Yvan Touitou, Alain Reinberg, David Touitou. Association between light at night, melatonin secretion, sleep deprivation, and the internal clock: Health impacts and mechanisms of circadian disruption. Life Sciences 2017. Vol. 173, 94-106.
47. Waterhouse, J; Reilly, T; Atkinson, G; Edwards. Jet lag: trends and coping strategies. The Lancet 2007. 369 (9567): 1117–1129.
48. Forbes-Robertson, S.; Dudley, E.; Vadgama, P.; Cook, C.; Drawer, S.; Kilduff, L. Circadian Disruption and Remedial Interventions. Sports Medicine 2012. 42 (3): 185–208.
49. Garaulet M, Gómez-Abellán P, Alburquerque-Béjar JJ, Lee YC, Ordovás JM, Scheer FA. Timing of food intake predicts weight loss effectiveness. Int J Obes (Lond). 2013.
50. Arble DM, Bass J, Laposky AD, Vitaterna MH, Turek FW. Circadian Timing of Food Intake Contributes to Weight Gain. Obesity. 2009. 17(11):2100–2102.
51. Hardeland R, Pandi-Perumal SR, Cardinali DP. Melatonin. The International Journal of Biochemistry & Cell Biology 2006. 38 (3): 313–16.
52. Arendt J, Skene DJ. Melatonin as a chronobiotic. Sleep Med Rev 2005. 9 (1): 25–39.
53. Espelund U, et al. Fasting unmasks a strong inverse association between ghrelin and cortisol in serum: studies in obese and normal-weight subjects. J Clin Endocrinol Metab. 2005. 90(2):741– 746.
54. Dzaja A, et al. Sleep enhances nocturnal plasma ghrelin levels in healthy subjects. Am J Physiol Endocrinol Metab. 2004. 286(6):E963–E967.
55. Shahrad Taheri, Ling Lin, Diane Austin, Terry Young and Emmanuel Mignot. Short Sleep Duration Is Associated with Reduced Leptin, Elevated Ghrelin, and Increased Body Mass Index. PLoS Med. 2004. 1(3): e62.
56. Czeisler, CA. Casting light on sleep deficiency. Nature 2013. Vol 497:S13.
57. Baron KG, Reid KJ, Kern AS, Zee PC. Role of sleep timing in caloric intake and BMI. Obesity (Silver Spring). 2011. 19(7):1374–1381.
58. Van Cauter E, Spiegel K, Tasali E, Leproult R. Metabolic consequences of sleep and sleep loss. Sleep Med. 2008. 9 Suppl 1:S23–28.
59. Cauter EV, et al. The Impact of Sleep Deprivation on Hormones and Metabolism. Medscape, 2005.
60. St-Onge MP, McReynolds A, Trivedi ZB, Roberts AL, Sy M, Hirsch J. Sleep restriction leads to increased activation of brain regions sensitive to food stimuli. Am J Clin Nutr. 2012. 95(4):818-24.

61. Mendlewicz J. Disruption of the circadian timing systems: molecular mechanisms in mood disorders. CNS Drugs. 2009. 23 Suppl 2:15–26.
62. Omar Mesarwi, MD, Jan Polak, Jonathan Jun, and Vsevolod Y. Polotsky. Sleep disorders and the development of insulin resistance and obesity. Endocrinol Metab Clin North Am. 2013. 42(3): 617–634.
63. Manuel D. Gahete José Córdoba-Chacón Qing Lin Jens C. Brüning C. Ronald Kahn Justo P. Castaño Helen Christian Raúl M. Luque Rhonda D. Kineman. Insulin and IGF-I Inhibit GH Synthesis and Release in Vitro and in Vivo by Separate Mechanisms. Endocrinology 2013. Vol. 154, I7, 2410–2420.
64. Eckhard Mühlbauer, Elke Albrecht, Kathleen Hofmann, Ivonne Bazwinsky-Wutschke, Elmar Peschke. Melatonin inhibits insulin secretion in rat insulinoma β-cells (INS-1) heterologously expressing the human melatonin receptor isoform MT2. Journal of Pineal Research 2011. Vol. 51, I3, 361-372.
65. Simon C, Gronfier C, Schlienger JL, Brandenberger G. Circadian and ultradian variations of leptin in normal man under continuous enteral nutrition: relationship to sleep and body temperature. J. Clin. Endocrinol. Metab. 1998; 83(6):1893–1899.
66. Kandil, T; Moussa, A; El-Gendy, AA; Abbas, AM. The potential therapeutic effect of melatonin in Gastro-Esohageal Reflux Disease. BMC Gastroenterology 2010. Review. BioMed Central. 10: 7.
67. Konturek PC, Brzozowski T, Konturek SJ. Gut clock: implication of circadian rhythms in the gastrointestinal tract. J Physiol Pharmacol. 2011. 62(2):139-50.
68. Asher G, Sassone-Corsi P. Time for food: the intimate interplay between nutrition, metabolism, and the circadian clock. Cell. 2015;161(1):84-92.
69. Ali T, Choe J, Awab A, et al. Sleep, immunity and inflammation in gastrointestinal disorders. World J Gastroenterol. 2013. 19(48):9231-9239.
70. Rosselot AE, Hong CI, Moore SR. Rhythm and bugs: circadian clocks, gut microbiota, and enteric infections. Curr Opin Gastroenterol. 2016;32(1):7-11.
71. Zarrinpar A, Chaix A, Yooseph S, Panda S. Diet and feeding pattern affect the diurnal dynamics of the gut microbiome. Cell Metab. 2014. 20(6):1006-17.
72. Tina M. Burke, Rachel R. Markwald1, Andrew W. McHill1, Evan D. Chinoy, Jesse A. Snider, Sara C. Bessman1, Christopher M. Jung1, John S. O'Neill and Kenneth P. Wright Jr. Effects of caffeine on the human circadian clock in vivo and in vitro. Science Translational Medicine 2015. Vol. 7, I305, 305ra146.

73. Scheer FA, et al. The human endogenous circadian system causes greatest platelet activation during the biological morning independent of behaviors. PLoS ONE. 2011; 6(9):e24549.
74. Mills E, Wu P, Seely D, Guyatt G. Melatonin in the treatment of cancer: a systematic review of randomized controlled trials and meta-analysis. J. Pineal Res 2005. 39 (4): 360–66.
75. Haus E, Smolensky M. Biological clocks and shift work: circadian dysregulation and potential long-term effects. Canc Causes Contr. 2006;17:489–500.
76. Davis S, Mirick DK, Stevens RG. Night shift work, light at night, and risk of breast cancer. J Natl Cancer Inst. 2001;93:1557–62.
77. Suwazono Y, Dochi M, Sakata K, et al. A longitudinal study on the effect of shift work on weight gain in male Japanese workers. Obesity (Silver Spring). 2008;16:1887–93.
78. Megumi Hatori, Christopher Vollmers, Amir Zarrinpar, Luciano DiTacchio, Eric A. Bushong, Shubhroz Gill, Mathias Leblanc, Amandine Chaix, Matthew Joens, James A.J. Fitzpatrick, Mark H. Ellisman and Satchidananda Panda. Time-restricted feeding without reducing caloric intake prevents metabolic diseases in mice fed a high-fat diet. Cell Metabolism 2012. 15(6):848-60
79. Sundaram S, Yan L. Time-restricted feeding reduces adiposity in mice fed a high-fat diet. Nutr Res. 2016. 36(6):603-11.
80. Duncan MJ, Smith JT, Narbaiza J, Mueez F, Bustle LB, Qureshi S, Fieseler C, Legan SJ. Restricting feeding to the active phase in middle-aged mice attenuates adverse metabolic effects of a high-fat diet. Physiol Behav. 2016. 167:1-9.
81. Chung H, Chou W, Sears DD, Patterson RE, Webster NJ, Ellies LG. Time-restricted feeding improves insulin resistance and hepatic steatosis in a mouse model of postmenopausal obesity. Metabolism. 2016. 65(12):1743-1754.
82. Rothschild J, Hoddy KK, Jambazian P, Varady KA. Time-restricted feeding and risk of metabolic disease: a review of human and animal studies. Nutr Rev. 2014. 72(5):308-18.
83. Tinsley GM, La Bounty PM. Effects of intermittent fasting on body composition and clinical health markers in humans. Nutr Rev. 2015. 73(10):661-74.
84. Stephen D. Anton, Keelin Moehl, William T. Donahoo, Krisztina Marosi, Stephanie A. Lee, Arch G. Mainous III, Christiaan Leeuwenburgh, Mark P. Mattson. Flipping the Metabolic Switch: Understanding and Applying the Health Benefits of Fasting. Obesity 2018. Vol. 26, I2, 254, 268.
85. Moro T, Tinsley G, Bianco A, Marcolin G, Pacelli QF, Battaglia G, Palma A, Gentil P, Neri M, Paoli A. Effects of eight weeks of time-restricted feeding (16/8) on basal metabolism, maximal strength, body composition,

inflammation, and cardiovascular risk factors in resistance-trained males. J Transl Med. 2016. 14(1):290.
86. Tinsley GM, Forsse JS, Butler NK, Paoli A, Bane AA, La Bounty PM, Morgan GB, Grandjean PW. Time-restricted feeding in young men performing resistance training: A randomized controlled trial. Eur J Sport Sci. 2017. 17(2):200-207.
87. Woodie LN, Luo Y, Wayne MJ, Graff EC, Ahmed B, O'Neill AM, Greene MW. Restricted feeding for 9h in the active period partially abrogates the detrimental metabolic effects of a Western diet with liquid sugar consumption in mice. Metabolism. 2018. 82:1-13.
88. Mattson MP, Longo VD, Harvie M. Impact of intermittent fasting on health and disease processes. Ageing Res Rev. 2017. 39:46-58.
89. Bayon V, Leger D, Gomez-Merino D, Vecchierini MF, Chennaoui M. Sleep debt and obesity. Ann Med. 2014. 46(5):264-72.
90. Amandine Chaix, Amir Zarrinpar, Phuong Miu and Satchidananda Panda. Time-restricted feeding is a preventative and therapeutic intervention against diverse nutritional challenges. Cell Metab. 2014. 20(6): 991–1005.
91. Bryan G. Allen, Sudershan K. Bhatia, Carryn M. Anderson, Julie M. Eichenberger-Gilmore, Zita A. Sibenaller, Kranti A. Mapuskar, Joshua D. Schoenfeld, John M. Buatti, Douglas R. Spitz, and Melissa A. Fath. Ketogenic diets as an adjuvant cancer therapy: History and potential mechanism. Redox Biol. 2014; 2: 963–970.
92. Branco AF, Ferreira A, Simões RF, Magalhães-Novais S, Zehowski C, Cope E, Silva AM, Pereira D, Sardão VA, Cunha-Oliveira T. Ketogenic diets: from cancer to mitochondrial diseases and beyond. Eur J Clin Invest. 2016 Mar;46(3):285-98.
93. Marinac CR, Nelson SH, Breen CI, Hartman SJ, Natarajan L, Pierce JP, Flatt SW, Sears DD, Patterson RE. Prolonged Nightly Fasting and Breast Cancer Prognosis. JAMA Oncol. 2016 Aug 1;2(8):1049-55.
94. Prof Marta Garaulet, Purificación Gómez-Abellán, Juan J Alburquerque-Béjar, Yu-Chi Lee, Prof Jose M Ordovás and Prof. Frank AJL Scheer. Timing of food intake predicts weight loss effectiveness. Int J Obes (Lond). 2013 Apr; 37(4): 604–611.
95. Anderson SE, Andridge R, Whitaker RC. Bedtime in Preschool-Aged Children and Risk for Adolescent Obesity. J Pediatr. 2016 Sep;176:17-22.
96. Arlet V. Nedeltcheva, Jennifer M. Kilkus, Jacqueline Imperial, Dale A. Schoeller and Plamen D. Penev. Insufficient sleep undermines dietary efforts to reduce adiposity. Ann Intern Med. 2010 Oct 5; 153(7): 435–441.
97. Magee L, Hale L. Longitudinal associations between sleep duration and subsequent weight gain: a systematic review. Sleep Med Rev. 2012 Jun;16(3):231-41.

98. Gill S, Panda S. A Smartphone App Reveals Erratic Diurnal Eating Patterns in Humans that Can Be Modulated for Health Benefits. Cell Metab. 2015 Nov 3;22(5):789-98.
99. Antoni R, Johnston KL, Collins AL, Robertson MD. Effects of intermittent fasting on glucose and lipid metabolism. Proc Nutr Soc. 2017 Aug;76(3):361-368.
100. Harvie MN, Howell T. Could Intermittent Energy Restriction and Intermittent Fasting Reduce Rates of Cancer in Obese, Overweight, and Normal-Weight Subjects? A Summary of Evidence. Adv Nutr. 2016 Jul 15;7(4):690-705.
101. Harvie MN, Pegington M, Mattson MP, Frystyk J, Dillon B, Evans G, Cuzick J, Jebb SA, Martin B, Cutler RG, Son TG, Maudsley S, Carlson OD, Egan JM, Flyvbjerg A, Howell A. The effects of intermittent or continuous energy restriction on weight loss and metabolic disease risk markers: a randomized trial in young overweight women. Int J Obes (Lond). 2011 May;35(5):714-27.
102. Antoni R, Johnston KL, Collins AL, Robertson MD. Intermittent v. continuous energy restriction: differential effects on postprandial glucose and lipid metabolism following matched weight loss in overweight/obese participants. Br J Nutr. 2018 Mar;119(5):507-516.
103. Gotthardt JD, Verpeut JL, Yeomans BL, et al. Intermittent fasting promotes fat loss with lean mass retention, increased hypothalamic norepinephrine content, and increased neuropeptide Y gene expression in diet-induced obese male mice. Endocrinology 2016;157:679-691.
104. Colman RJ, Anderson RM, Johnson SC, et al. Caloric restriction delays disease onset and mortality in rhesus monkeys. Science 2009;325:201-204.
105. Redman LM, Ravussin E. Caloric restriction in humans: impact on physiological, psychological, and behavioral outcomes. Antioxid Redox Signal 2011;14:275-287.
106. Anton S, Leeuwenburgh C. Fasting or caloric restriction for healthy aging. Exp Gerontol 2013;48:1003-1005.
107. Harvie M, Wright C, Pegington M, et al. The effect of intermittent energy and carbohydrate restriction v. daily energy restriction on weight loss and metabolic disease risk markers in overweight women. Br J Nutr 2013;110:1534-1547.
108. Tadahiro Shimazu, Matthew D. Hirschey, John Newman, Wenjuan He, Kotaro Shirakawa, Natacha Le Moan, Carrie A. Grueter, Hyungwook Lim, Laura R. Saunders, Robert D. Stevens, Christopher B. Newgard, Robert V. Farese, Jr., Rafael de Cabo, Scott Ulrich, Katerina Akassoglou and Eric Verdin. Suppression of Oxidative Stress by β-Hydroxybutyrate, an Endogenous Histone Deacetylase Inhibitor. Science. 2013 Jan 11; 339(6116): 211–214.

109. Hirschey MD, Shimazu T, Goetzman E, et al. SIRT3 regulates mitochondrial fatty-acid oxidation by reversible enzyme deacetylation. Nature 2010;464:121-125.
110. Shimazu T, Hirschey MD, Hua L, et al. SIRT3 deacetylates mitochondrial 3-hydroxy-3-methylglutaryl CoA synthase 2 and regulates ketone body production. Cell Metab 2010;12:654-661.
111. Nadia Aalling Jessen, Anne Sofie Finmann, MunkIben Lundgaard, Maiken Nedergaard. The Glymphatic System: A Beginner's Guide. Neurochemical Research 2015. Vol. 40, I12, 2583–2599.
112. Iliff JJ, Nedergaard M. Is there a cerebral lymphatic system? Stroke 2013. 44:S93–S95.
113. Xie L, Kang H, Xu Q et al. Sleep drives metabolite clearance from the adult brain. Science 2013. 342:373–377.
114. Canto C, Jiang LQ, Deshmukh AS, et al. Interdependence of AMPK and SIRT1 for metabolic adaptation to fasting and exercise in skeletal muscle. Cell Metab 2010;11:213-219.
115. Puchalska P, Crawford PA. Multi-dimensional roles of ketone bodies in fuel metabolism, signaling, and therapeutics. Cell Metab 2017;25:262-284.
116. Morris CJ, Yang JN, Scheer FA. The impact of the circadian timing system on cardiovascular and metabolic function. Prog Brain Res. 2012; 199:337-58.
117. Rachel R. Markwald, Edward L. Melanson, Mark R. Smith, Janine Higgins, Leigh Perreault, Robert H. Eckel and Kenneth P. Wright, Jr.. Impact of insufficient sleep on total daily energy expenditure, food intake, and weight gain. Proc Natl Acad Sci U S A. 2013 Apr 2; 110(14): 5695–5700.
118. Marie-Pierre St-Onge. The Role of Sleep Duration in the Regulation of Energy Balance: Effects on Energy Intakes and Expenditure. J Clin Sleep Med. 2013 Jan 15; 9(1): 73–80.
119. Yasumoto Y, Hashimoto C, Nakao R, Yamazaki H, Hiroyama H, Nemoto T, Yamamoto S, Sakurai M, Oike H, Wada N, Yoshida-Noro C, Oishi K. Short-term feeding at the wrong time is sufficient to desynchronize peripheral clocks and induce obesity with hyperphagia, physical inactivity and metabolic disorders in mice. Metabolism. 2016 May;65(5):714-27.
120. Valter D. Longo and Satchidananda Panda. Fasting, Circadian Rhythms, and Time-Restricted Feeding in Healthy Lifespan. Cell Metabolism 2016. 23.
121. Valter D. Longo and Mark P. Mattson. Fasting: Molecular Mechanisms and Clinical Applications. Cell Metab. 2014 February 4; 19(2): 181–192.
122. Jakubowicz D, Barnea M, Wainstein J, Froy O. High caloric intake at breakfast vs. dinner differentially influences weight loss of overweight and obese women. Obesity (Silver Spring) 2013. 21(12): 2504–2512.

123. Iriti M, Varoni EM, Vitalini S. Melatonin in traditional Mediterranean diets. Journal of Pineal Research 2010. 49 (2): 101–05.
124. Reiter RJ, Manchester LC, Tan DX. Melatonin in walnuts: influence on levels of melatonin and total antioxidant capacity of blood. Nutrition 2005. 21 (9): 920–24.
125. Lee, C., and Longo, V.D. Fasting vs dietary restriction in cellular protection and cancer treatment: from model organisms to patients. Oncogene 2011. 30, 3305–3316.
126. Di Ma, Satchidananda Panda, Jiandie D Lin. Temporal orchestration of circadian autophagy rhythm by C/EBPβ. The EMBO Journal 2011. 30, 4642-4651.
127. Neuberger J. Surgery: Day or night--does the time of liver transplantation matter? Nature Reviews. Gastroenterology & Hepatology 2010. 7(11):596-597.

Chapter Two – Mindset

1. Schwartz MW, Woods SC, Porte D Jr, Seeley RJ, Baskin DG. Central nervous system control of food intake. Nature 2000; 404:661–671
2. Wilding JP. Neuropeptides and appetite control. Diabet Med 2002 ; 19(8):619-27.
3. Ahima RS, Antwi DA. Brain regulation of appetite and satiety. Endocrinol Metab Clin North Am 2008. Dec; 37(4): 811–823.
4. Cameron JD, Cyr MJ, Doucet E. Increased meal frequency does not promote greater weight loss in subjects who were prescribed an 8-week equi-energetic energy-restricted diet. Br J Nutr 2010. Apr;103(8):1098-101.
5. Williams G, Bing C, Cai XJ, Harrold JA, King PJ, Liu XH. The hypothalamus and the control of energy homeostasis: different circuits, different purposes. Physiol Behav. 2001 Nov-Dec;74(4-5):683-701.
6. Broberger C, Hokfelt T. Hypothalamic and vagal neuropeptide circuitries regulating food intake. Physiol Behav 2001. 74:669–682
7. George WM Millington. The role of proopiomelanocortin (POMC) neurones in feeding behaviour. Nutr Metab (Lond). 2007; 4: 18.
8. Balthasar N, Coppari R, McMinn J et al. Leptin receptor signaling in POMC neurons is required for normal body weight homeostasis. Neuron 2004; 42: 983–991.
9. MacNeil DJ, Howard AD, Guan X, Fong TM, Nargund RP, Bednarek MA, Goulet MT, Weinberg DH, Strack AM, Marsh DJ, Chen HY, Shen CP, Chen AS, Rosenblum CI, MacNeil T, Tota M, MacIntyre ED, Van der Ploeg LH. The role of melanocortins in body weight

regulation: opportunities for the treatment of obesity. Eur J Pharmacol. 2002 Aug 16;450(1):93-109.
10. Rogge G, Jones D, Hubert GW, Lin Y, Kuhar MJ.). CART peptides: regulators of body weight, reward and other functions. Nature Reviews. Neuroscience 2008. 9 (10): 747–58.
11. Zhang M, Han L, Xu Y. Roles of cocaine- and amphetamine-regulated transcript in the central nervous system. Clin. Exp. Pharmacol. Physiol 2011. 39 (6): 586–92.
12. Upadhya MA, Nakhate KT, Kokare DM, Singh U, Singru PS, Subhedar NK. CART peptide in the nucleus accumbens shell acts downstream to dopamine and mediates the reward and reinforcement actions of morphine. Neuropharmacology 2012. 62 (4): 1823–33.
13. Dandekar MP, Singru PS, Kokare DM, Lechan RM, Thim L, Clausen JT, Subhedar NK. Importance of cocaine- and amphetamine-regulated transcript peptide in the central nucleus of amygdala in anxiogenic responses induced by ethanol withdrawal. Neuropsychopharmacology 2008. 33 (5): 1127–36.
14. Kuo LE, Kitlinska JB, Tilan JU, Li L, Baker SB, Johnson MD, Lee EW, Burnett MS, Fricke ST, Kvetnansky R, Herzog H, Zukowska Z. Neuropeptide Y acts directly in the periphery on fat tissue and mediates stress-induced obesity and metabolic syndrome. Nature Medicine 2007. 13 (7): 803–11.
15. Minor RK, Chang JW, de Cabo R. Hungry for life: How the arcuate nucleus and neuropeptide Y may play a critical role in mediating the benefits of calorie restriction. Molecular and Cellular Endocrinology 2009. 299 (1): 79–88.
16. Pablo J. Enriori Anne E. Evans Puspha Sinnayah Michael A. Cowley. Leptin Resistance and Obesity. Obesity 2006. 14, S8, 254S-258S
17. Fekete C, Sarkar S, Rand WM, Harney JW, Emerson CH, Bianco AC, Lechan RM. Agouti-related protein (AGRP) has a central inhibitory action on the hypothalamic-pituitary-thyroid (HPT) axis; comparisons between the effect of AGRP and neuropeptide Y on energy homeostasis and the HPT axis. Endocrinology 2002. Oct;143(10):3846-53.
18. Inutsuka, A., Inui, A., Tabuchi, S., Tsunematsu, T., Lazarus, M., and Yamanaka, A.. Concurrent and robust regulation of feeding behaviors and metabolism by orexin neurons. Neuropharmacology 2014. 85, 451–460.
19. J. E., Chen, J., Tang, J. Y., Lehnert, H., Matthews, R. N., and Randeva, H. S.. Orexin receptor expression in human adipose tissue: effects of orexin-A and orexin-B. J. Endocrinol 2006. 191, 129–136.

20. Teske, J., Perez-Leighton, C., Billington, C., and Kotz, C.. Role of the locus coeruleus in enhanced orexin A-induced spontaneous physical activity in obesity-resistant rats. Am. J. Physiol. Regul. Integr. Comp. Physiol 2013. 305, R1337– R1345.
21. Thorpe, A. J., and Kotz, C. M.. Orexin A in the nucleus accumbens stimulates feeding and locomotor activity. Brain Res 2005. 1050, 156–162.
22. Hasegawa, E., Yanagisawa, M., Sakurai, T., and Mieda, M. Orexin neurons suppress narcolepsy via 2 distinct efferent pathways. J. Clin. Invest 2014. 124, 604–616.
23. Nishino, S., Ripley, B., Overeem, S., Lammers, G. J., and Mignot, E.. Hypocretin (orexin) deficiency in human narcolepsy. Lancet 2000. 355, 39–40.
24. Heier, M. S., Jansson, T. S., and Gautvik, K. M. Cerebrospinal fluid hypocretin 1 deficiency, overweight and metabolic dysregulation in patients with narcolepsy. J. Clin. Sleep Med 2011. 7, 653–658.
25. Harris, G., and Aston-Jones, G. Arousal and reward: a dichotomy in orexin function. Trends Neurosci 2006. 29, 571–577.
26. Lutter M, Krishnan V, Russo SJ, Jung S, McClung CA, Nestler EJ. Orexin signaling mediates the antidepressant-like effect of calorie restriction. J Neurosci. 2008 Mar 19;28(12):3071-5.
27. Harris GC, Wimmer M, Aston-Jones G. A role for lateral hypothalamic orexin neurons in reward seeking. Nature 2005; 437: 556–559.
28. Novak, C. M., and Levine, J. A. Daily intra-paraventricular Orexin-A treatment induces weight loss in rats. Obesity (Silver Spring) 2010. 17, 1493–1498.
29. Sellayah, D., Bharaj, P., and Sikder, D. Orexin is required for brown adipose tissue development, differentiation and function. Cell Metab. 2011. 14, 478– 490.
30. Teske, J. A., Billington, C. J., and Kotz, C. M. Hypocretin/orexin and energy expenditure. Acta Physiol. (Oxf.) 2010. 198, 303–312.
31. Antal-Zimanyi, I. Khawaja, X. The Role of Melanin-Concentrating Hormone in Energy Homeostasis and Mood Disorders. J Mol Neurosci 2009. 39: 1-2. 86-98.
32. Wren AM, Seal LJ, Cohen MA, Brynes AE, Frost GS, Murphy KG, Dhillo WS, Ghatei MA, Bloom SR. Ghrelin enhances appetite and increases food intake in humans. J Clin Endocrinol Metab 2001. 86:5992
33. English PJ, Ghatei MA, Malik IA, Bloom SR, Wilding JP. Food fails to suppress ghrelin levels in obese humans. J Clin Endocrinol Metab 2002. 87:2984.

34. Hansen TK, Dall R, Hosoda H, Kojima M, Kangawa K, Christiansen JS, Jorgensen JO. Weight loss increases circulating levels of ghrelin in human obesity. Clin Endocrinol (Oxf) 2002. 56:203–206.
35. Muyesser Sayki Arslan, Oya Topaloglu, Melia Karakose, Bekir Ucan, Esra Tutal, Basak Karbek, Ilknur Ozturk Unsal, Askin Gungunes, Taner Demirci, Mustafa Caliskan, Zeynep Ginis, Mustafa Sahin, Erman Cakal, Mustafa Ozbek, Tuncay Delibasi. Ghrelin may have a role in obesity pathogenesis in patients with vitamin D deficiency. Endocrine Abstracts 2014. 35 P139.
36. Dickson SL, Egecioglu E, Landgren S, Skibicka KP, Engel JA, Jerlhag E. The role of the central ghrelin system in reward from food and chemical drugs. Molecular and Cellular Endocrinology 2011. 340 (1): 80–87.
37. Karen E. Foster-Schubert, Joost Overduin, Catherine E. Prudom, Jianhua Liu, Holly S. Callahan, Bruce D. Gaylinn, Michael O. Thorner, David E. Cummings. Acyl and Total Ghrelin Are Suppressed Strongly by Ingested Proteins, Weakly by Lipids, and Biphasically by Carbohydrates. The Journal of Clinical Endocrinology & Metabolism 2008. Vol. 93, I5, 1971–1979.
38. L. Sominsky, A. Soch, I. Ziko, S.N. De Luca, M.R. Di Natale, S.J.Spencer. Ghrelin – a novel link between stress and infertility. Brain, Behavior, and Immunity 2017. Vol. 66, S, e22.
39. Lutter M, Sakata I, Osborne-Lawrence S, Rovinsky SA, Anderson JG, Jung S, Birnbaum S, Yanagisawa M, Elmquist JK, Nestler EJ, Zigman JM. The orexigenic hormone ghrelin defends against depressive symptoms of chronic stress. Nature Neuroscience 2008. 11 (7): 752–53.
40. K. Simpson, J. Parker, J. Plumer, S. Bloom. CCK, PYY and PP: The Control of Energy Balance. Appetite Control 2011. pp 209-230.
41. Batterham RL, Le Roux CW, Cohen MA, Park AJ, Ellis SM, Patterson M, Frost GS, Ghatei MA, Bloom SR. Pancreatic polypeptide reduces appetite and food intake in humans. J Clin Endocrinol Metab 2003. 88:3989–3992.
42. Batterham RL, Le Roux CW, Cohen MA, Park AJ, Ellis SM, Patterson M, Frost GS, Ghatei MA, Bloom SR. Pancreatic polypeptide reduces appetite and food intake in humans. J Clin Endocrinol Metab 2003. 88:3989–3992.
43. Batterham RL, Bloom SR. The gut hormone peptide YY regulates appetite. Ann NY Acad Sci 2003. 994:162–168.
44. Gundula R. R. Kiess, Reinhold G. Laessle. Stress inhibits PYY secretion in obese and normal weight women. Eating and Weight Disorders - Studies on Anorexia, Bulimia and Obesity 2016. Vol 21, I2, 245-249.

45. Meier JJ, Gallwitz B, Schmidt WE, Nauck MA. Glucagon-like peptide 1 as a regulator of food intake and body weight: therapeutic perspectives. Eur J Pharmacol 2002. 440:269–279.
46. Flint A , Raben A , Ersboll AK , Holst JJ , Astrup A. The effect of physiological levels of glucagon-like peptide-1 on appetite, gastric emptying, energy and substrate metabolism in obesity. Int J Obes Relat Metab Disord 2001. 25:781–792.
47. Juhl CB, Hollingdal M , Sturis J , Jakobsen G , Agerso H , Veldhuis J, Porksen N , Schmitz O. Bedtime administration of NN2211, a long-acting GLP-1 derivative, substantially reduces fasting and postprandial glycemia in type 2 diabetes. Diabetes 2002. 51:424–429.
48. Cohen MA, Ellis SM , Le Roux CW , Batterham RL , Park A , Patterson M , Frost GS , Ghatei MA , Bloom SR. Oxyntomodulin suppresses appetite and reduces food intake in humans. J Clin Endocrinol Metab 2003. 88:4696–4701.
49. Wilcox G. Insulin and insulin resistance. The Clinical Biochemist 2005. Reviews. 26 (2): 19–39.
50. Christine Dalgård, Maria Skaalum Petersen, Pal Weihe, Philippe Grandjean. Vitamin D Status in Relation to Glucose Metabolism and Type 2 Diabetes in Septuagenarians. Diabetes Care 2011. Jun; 34(6): 1284-1288.
51. Coll AP, Farooqi IS, O'Rahilly S. The hormonal control of food intake. Cell 2007; 129: 251–262.
52. Scarpace PJ, Zhang Y. Leptin resistance: a predisposing factor for diet-induced obesity. Am J Physiol Regul Integr Comp Physiol 2009; 296: R493–R500.
53. Myers MG Jr, Leibel RL, Seeley RJ, Schwartz MW. Obesity and leptin resistance: Distinguishing cause from effect. Trends Endocrinol Metab. 2010. 21(11):643-51.
54. Enriori PJ, Evans AE, Sinnayah P, Jobst EE, Tonelli-Lemos L, Billes SK, Glavas MM, Grayson BE, Perello M, Nillni EA, Grove KL, Cowley MA. Diet-induced obesity causes severe but reversible leptin resistance in arcuate melanocortin neurons. Cell Metabolism 2007. 5 (3): 181–94.
55. Kieffer TJ, Damond N, Herrera PL. Insulin and Glucagon: Partners for Life. Endocrinology 2017. 158 (4): 696–701.
56. Jones BJ, Tan T, Bloom SR. Minireview: Glucagon in stress and energy homeostasis. Endocrinology 2012. 153 (3): 1049–54.
57. Vuddanda PR, Chakraborty S, Singh S. Berberine: a potential phytochemical with multispectrum therapeutic activities. Expert Opin Investig Drugs. (2010)
58. B. Vandanmagsar K. R. Haynie S. E. Wicks E. M. Bermudez T. M. Mendoza D. Ribnicky W. T. Cefalu R. L. Mynatt. Artemisia

dracunculus L. extract ameliorates insulin sensitivity by attenuating inflammatory signalling in human skeletal muscle culture. Diabetes, Obesity and Metabolism 2014. Vol. 16, I8.
59. Huyen VT, Phan DV, Thang P, Hoa NK, Ostenson CG. Antidiabetic effect of Gynostemma pentaphyllum tea in randomly assigned type 2 diabetic patients. Horm Metab Res. 2010. 42(5):353-7.
60. Ringseis R, Keller J, Eder K. Role of carnitine in the regulation of glucose homeostasis and insulin sensitivity: evidence from in vivo and in vitro studies with carnitine supplementation and carnitine deficiency. Eur J Nutr. 2012. 51(1):1-18.
61. Wang GJ, Tomasi D, Backus W, Wang R, Telang F, Geliebter A, Korner J, Bauman A, Fowler JS, Thanos PK, Volkow ND. Gastric distention activates satiety circuitry in the human brain. Neuroimage. 2008 Feb 15;39(4):1824-31. Epub 2007 Nov 22.
62. Gannon MC, Nuttall FQ. Effect of a high-protein diet on ghrelin, growth hormone, and insulin-like growth factor-I and binding proteins 1 and 3 in subjects with type 2 diabetes mellitus. Metabolism. 2011 Sep;60(9):1300-11.
63. Blom WA, Lluch A, Stafleu A, Vinoy S, Holst JJ, Schaafsma G, Hendriks HF. Effect of a high-protein breakfast on the postprandial ghrelin response. Am J Clin Nutr. 2006 Feb;83(2):211-20.
64. Spiegel K, Tasali E, Penev P, Van Cauter E. Brief communication: Sleep curtailment in healthy young men is associated with decreased leptin levels, elevated ghrelin levels, and increased hunger and appetite. Ann Intern Med. 2004. 141(11):846-50.
65. Hannah Greenwood, Anne McGavigan, Mohammad Ghatei, Stephen Bloom & Kevin Murphy. The effect of specific micronutrients on appetite. Endocrine Abstracts 2012. 28 P170.
66. Gianini, L.M., White, M.A., Masheb, R.M. Eating pathology, emotion regulation, and emotional overeating in obese adults with binge eating disorder. Eating Behaviors 2013. Vol. 14, I3, 309-313.
67. Leehu Zysberg. Emotional intelligence, anxiety, and emotional eating: A deeper insight into a recently reported association? Eating Behaviors 2018. Vol. 29, 128-131.
68. Feinstein, Justin S.; Adolphs, Ralph; Damasio, Antonio; Tranel, Daniel. The Human Amygdala and the Induction and Experience of Fear. Current Biology 2011. 21 (1): 34–8.
69. Paré D., Collins D.R., Pelletier J.G. Amygdala oscillations and the consolidation of emotional memories. Trends in Cognitive Sciences 2002. 6 (7): 306–314.
70. Torres S.T. and Nowson C.A. Relationship between stress, eating behavior and obesity. Nutrition 2007; 23 (11-12): 887-94.

71. Tanja C. Adam, Elissa S. Epel. Stress, eating and the reward system. Physiology & Behavior 2007. 91, 449–458.
72. Elissa Epel, Rachel Lapidus, Bruce McEwen, Kelly Brownell. Stress may add bite to appetite in women: a laboratory study of stress-induced cortisol and eating behaviour. Psychoneuroendocrinology 2001. 26, 37–49
73. Stice E, Yokum S, Zald D, Dagher A. Dopamine-based reward circuitry responsivity, genetics, and overeating. Curr Top Behav Neurosci. 2011. 6:81-93.
74. Wang GJ, Volkow ND, Fowler JS. The role of dopamine in motivation for food in humans: implications for obesity. Expert Opin Ther Targets. 2002 Oct;6(5):601-9.
75. Volkow N. D.; Wang G. J.; Fowler J. S.; Telang F. Overlapping neuronal circuits in addiction and obesity: Evidence of systems pathology. Philos. Trans. R. Soc. 2008. B 363, 3191–3200.
76. David J Mysels and Maria A Sullivan. The relationship between opioid and sugar intake: Review of evidence and clinical applications. J Opioid Manag. 2010 Nov-Dec; 6(6): 445–452.
77. Jetro J. Tuulari, Lauri Tuominen, Femke E. de Boer, Jussi Hirvonen, Semi Helin, Pirjo Nuutila, Lauri Nummenmaa. Feeding Releases Endogenous Opioids in Humans. The Journal of Neuroscience, 2017; 37 (34): 8284
78. Halford, JC et al. Serotonin (5-HT) drugs: effects on appetite suppression and use for the treatment of obesity. Current drug targets 2005, 6(2): 201-213.
79. Figlewicz DP, Naleid A MacDonald, Sipols AJ. Modulation of food reward by adiposity signals. Physiol Behav 2007; 91: 473–478.
80. Fulton S, Pissios P, Manchon RP et al. Leptin regulation of the mesoaccumbens dopamine pathway. Neuron 2006; 51: 811–822.
81. Hommel JD, Trinko R, Sears RM et al. Leptin receptor signaling in midbrain dopamine neurons regulates feeding. Neuron 2006; 51: 801–810.
82. Paul M Johnson, Paul J Kenny. Dopamine D2 receptors in addiction-like reward dysfunction and compulsive eating in obese rats. Nature Neuroscience, 2010.
83. Xin-Yun Lu. The leptin hypothesis of depression: a potential link between mood disorders and obesity? Curr Opin Pharmacol. 2007 Dec; 7(6): 648–652.
84. Charnay Y, Cusin I, Vallet PG, Muzzin P, Rohner-Jeanrenaud F, Bouras C. Intracerebroventricular infusion of leptin decreases serotonin transporter binding sites in the frontal cortex of the rat. Neurosci Lett. 2000 Apr 7; 283(2):89-92.

85. Lu XY, Kim CS, Frazer A, Zhang W. Leptin: a potential novel antidepressant. Proc Natl Acad Sci U S A. 2006. 103:1593–1598.
86. Gimpl G, Fahrenholz F. The oxytocin receptor system: structure, function, and regulation. Physiological Reviews 2001. 81 (2): 629–83.
87. Lee HJ, Macbeth AH, Pagani JH, Young WS. Oxytocin: the great facilitator of life. Progress in Neurobiology 2009. 88 (2): 127–51.
88. Kalm, Leah, and Richard D. Semba. They Starved So That Others Be Better Fed: Remembering Ancel Keys and the Minnesota Experiment. JN: The Journal of Nutrition 2005. 135, No. 6: 1347–1352.
89. Tucker, Todd. The Great Starvation Experiment: Ancel Keys and the Men Who Starved for Science. Minneapolis: University of Minnesota Press, 2006.
90. Thomas DM, Bouchard C, Church T, et al. Why do individuals not lose more weight from an exercise intervention at a defined dose? An energy balance analysis. Obes Rev 2012. 13:835–847
91. Swift D, Johannsen N, Lavie C, Earnest C, Church T. The role of exercise and physical activity in weight loss and maintenance. Prog Cardiovasc Dis 2014. 56:441–447
92. Arcelus, J; Witcomb, GL; Mitchell, A. Prevalence of eating disorders amongst dancers: a systemic review and meta-analysis. European Eating Disorders Review 2014. 22 (2): 92–101.
93. Harrison, Kristen. Ourselves, Our Bodies: Thin-Ideal Media, Self-Discrepancies, and Eating Disorder Symptomatology in Adolescents. Journal of Social and Clinical Psychology 2001. 20 (3): 289–323.
94. Swinbourne, JM; Touyz, SW. The co-morbidity of eating disorders and anxiety disorders: a review. European Eating Disorders Review 2007. 15 (4): 253–74.
95. Fox, John. Eating Disorders and Emotions. Clinical Psychology & Psychotherapy 2009. 16 (237–239): 237–239.
96. Jane A.Foster, Linda Rinaman, John F.Cryan. Stress & the gut-brain axis: Regulation by the microbiome. Neurobiology of Stress 2017. Vol. 7, 124-136.
    A. Bharwani, M.F. Mian, J.A. Foster, M.G. Surette, J. Bienenstock, P. Forsythe. Structural & functional consequences of chronic psychosocial stress on the microbiome & host. Psychoneuroendocrinology 2016. 63, pp. 217-227.
97. M.G. Gareau. Microbiota-gut-brain axis and cognitive function. Adv. Exp. Med. Biol. 2014. 817, pp. 357-371.
98. B.E. Leonard. HPA and immune axes in stress: involvement of the serotonergic system. Neuroimmunomodulat 2006. 13, pp. 268-276.

99. K. Schmidt, P.J. Cowen, C.J. Harmer, G. Tzortzis, S. Errington, P.W. Burnet. Prebiotic intake reduces the waking cortisol response and alters emotional bias in healthy volunteers. Psychopharmacology 2015. 232, pp. 1793-1801.
100. A.P. Allen, W. Hutch, Y.E. Borre, P.J. Kennedy, A. Temko, G. Boylan, E. Murphy, J.F. Cryan, T.G. Dinan, G. Clarke. Bifidobacterium longum 1714 as a translational psychobiotic: modulation of stress, electrophysiology and neurocognition in healthy volunteers. Transl. Psychiatry 2016. 6.
101. Barry E. Levin. The drive to regain is mainly in the brain. Am J Physiol Regul Integr Comp Physiol 2004. 287: R1297–R1300.
102. MacLean PS, Higgins JA, Johnson GC, Fleming-Elder BK, Peters JC, and Hill JO. Metabolic adjustments with the development, treatment, and recurrence of obesity in obesity-prone rats. Am J Physiol Regul Integr Comp Physiol 2004. 287: R288–R297.
103. Lipton BH. The Biology of Belief. Hay House 2005.
104. Tapper, K., Shaw, C., Ilsley, J., et al. Exploratory randomised controlled trial of a mindfulness based weight loss intervention for women. Appetite 2008.
105. Linardon, Jake; Wade, Tracey D.; Garcia, Xochitl de la Piedad; Brennan, Leah. The efficacy of cognitive-behavioral therapy for eating disorders: A systematic review and meta-analysis. Journal of Consulting and Clinical Psychology 2017. 85 (11): 1080–1094.
106. McKay D, Sookman D, Neziroglu F, Wilhelm S, Stein DJ, Kyrios M, Matthews K, Veale D. Efficacy of cognitive-behavioral therapy for obsessive-compulsive disorder. Psychiatry Research 2015. 225 (3): 236–246.
107. Shawn N.Katterman, Brighid M. Kleinman, Megan M. Hood, Lisa M. Nackers, Joyce A. Corsica. Mindfulness meditation as an intervention for binge eating, emotional eating, and weight loss: A systematic review. Eating Behaviors 2014. Vol. 15, I2, 197-204.
108. Thoma MV, La Marca R, Brönnimann R, Finkel L, Ehlert U, Nater UM. The Effect of Music on the Human Stress Response. PLoS ONE 2013. 8(8): e70156.
109. Taheri S. The link between short sleep duration and obesity: we should recommend more sleep to prevent obesity. Arch Dis Child. 2006. 91(11):881– 884.
110. Cristiana Duarte, José Pinto-Gouveia. The impact of early shame memories in Binge Eating Disorder: The mediator effect of current body image shame and cognitive fusion. Psychiatry Research 2017. Vol. 258, 511-517.
111. Cristiana Duarte, Cláudia Ferreira, José Pinto-Gouveia. At the core of eating disorders: Overvaluation, social rank, self-criticism and shame

in anorexia, bulimia and binge eating disorder. Comprehensive Psychiatry 2016. Vol. 66, 123-131.
112. Mara Iannaccone, Francesca D'Olimpio, Stefania Cella, Paolo Cotrufo. Self-esteem, body shame and eating disorder risk in obese and normal weight adolescents: A mediation model. Eating Behaviors 2016. Vol. 21, 80-83.
113. Cristiana Duarte, José Pinto-Gouveia, Cláudia Ferreira. Escaping from body image shame and harsh self-criticism: Exploration of underlying mechanisms of binge eating. Eating Behaviors 2014. Vol. 15, I4, 638-643.
114. Inge Brechan, Ingela Lundin Kvalem. Relationship between body dissatisfaction and disordered eating: Mediating role of self-esteem and depression. Eating Behaviors 2015. Vol. 17, 49-58.
115. David CA, Levitan RD, Reid C, Carter JC, Kaplan AS, Patte KA, King N, Curtis C, Kenedy JL. Dopamine for 'wanting' and opioids for 'liking': a comparison of obese adults with and without binge eating. Obesity. 2009. 17(6):1220–1225.
116. Serena D Stevens, Sylvia Herbozo, Holly ER Morrell, Lauren M Schaefer and J Kevin Thompson, Adult and childhood weight influence body image and depression through weight stigmatization, Journal of Health Psychology 2017. 22, 8, (1084).
117. Jessica M.Murakami, Jamal H.Essayli, Janet D.Latner. The relative stigmatization of eating disorders and obesity in males and females. Appetite 2016. Vol. 102, 77-82.
118. Lenny R.Vartanianm Alexis M.Porter. Weight stigma and eating behavior: A review of the literature. Appetite 2016. Vol. 102, 3-14.
119. Soh, NL; Touyz, SW; Surgenor, LJ. Eating and body image disturbances across cultures: A review. European Eating Disorders Review 2006. 14 (1): 54–65.
120. Laura Salerno, Gianluca Lo Coco, Salvatore Gullo, Rosalia Iacoponelli, Marie Louise Caltabiano and Lina A. Ricciardelli. Self-esteem mediates the associations among negative affect, body disturbances, and interpersonal problems in treatment-seeking obese individuals. Clinical Psychologist 2014. 19, 2, (85-95).
121. Martha Peaslee Levine. Loneliness and Eating Disorders. The Journal of Psychology 2012. 146, 1-2, (243).
122. Makiko Nakade, Naomi Aiba, Akemi Morita, Motohiko Miyachi, Satoshi Sasaki, and Shaw Watanabe. What Behaviors Are Important for Successful Weight Maintenance? Journal of Obesity 2012.
123. Cole R, Horacek T: Effectiveness of the "My Body Knows When" intuitive- eating pilot program. Am J Health Behav 2010. 34:286-297.

124. Weigensberg M, Shoar Z, Lane C, Spruijt-Metz D: Intuitive eating (IE) Is associated with decreased adiposity and increased insulin sensitivity (Si) in obese Latina female adolescents. DiabetesPro 2009.
125. Feng Wang, Heather M. Orpana, Howard Morrison, Margaret de Groh, Sulan Dai, Wei Luo. Long-term Association Between Leisure-time Physical Activity and Changes in Happiness: Analysis of the Prospective National Population Health Survey. American Journal of Epidemiology 2012. Vol. 176, I12, 1095–1100.

Chapter Three – Nutrition

1. Margaret E. Smith, Dion G. Morton. The Digestive System. Churchill Livingstone 2010.
2. Kong F, Singh RP. Disintegration of solid foods in human stomach. J. Food Sci 2008. 73 (5): R67–80.
3. Stiegler P, Cunliffe A. The role of diet and exercise for the maintenance of fat-free mass and resting metabolic rate during weight loss. Sports Medicine 2006. 36 (3): 239–262.
4. Johnstone AM, Murison SD, Duncan JS, Rance KA, Speakman JR, Koh YO. Factors influencing variation in basal metabolic rate include fat-free mass, fat mass, age, and circulating thyroxine but not sex, circulating leptin, or triiodothyronine. American Journal of Clinical Nutrition 2005. 82 (5): 941–948.
5. Pratley, R; Nicklas, B; Rubin, M; Miller, J; Smith, A; Smith, M; Hurley, B; Goldberg, A. Strength training increases resting metabolic rate and norepinephrine levels in healthy 50- to 65-year-old men. Journal of Applied Physiology 1994. 76 (1): 133–137.
6. Grattan BJ Jr; Connolly-Schoonen J. Addressing weight loss recidivism: a clinical focus on metabolic rate and the psychological aspects of obesity. ISRN Obesity. 2012: 567530.
7. Tsai, AG; Wadden, TA. Systematic review: An evaluation of major commercial weight loss programs in the United States. Annals of Internal Medicine 2005. 142 (1): 56–66.
8. Carla E. Cox. Role of Physical Activity for Weight Loss and Weight Maintenance. Diabetes Spectrum 2017. 30(3): 157-160.
9. Polak J, Klimcakova E, Moro C, Viguerie N, Berlan M, Hejnova J, Richterova B, Kraus I, Langin D, Stich V. Effect of aerobic training on plasma levels and subcutaneous abdominal adipose tissue gene expression of adiponectin, leptin, interleukin 6, and tumor necrosis factor alpha in obese women. Metabolism. 2006 Oct;55(10):1375-81.
10. Javier T. Gonzalez, Rachel C. Veasey, Penny L. S. Rumbold, Emma J. Stevenson. Breakfast and exercise contingently affect postprandial

metabolism and energy balance in physically active males. British Journal of Nutrition, 2013; 1.
11. Egan B, Zierath JR. Exercise metabolism and the molecular regulation of skeletal muscle adaptation. Cell Metabolism 2013. 17 (2): 162–184.
12. Basso JC, Suzuki WA. The Effects of Acute Exercise on Mood, Cognition, Neurophysiology, and Neurochemical Pathways: A Review. Brain Plasticity 2017. 2 (2): 127–152.
13. Halton, T. L., & Hu, F. B. The effects of high protein diets on thermogenesis, satiety and weight loss: a critical review. Journal of the American College of Nutrition 2004, 23(5), 373e385.
14. Peter Aldiss, James Betts, Craig Sale, Mark Pope, Helen Budge, Michael E. Symonds. Mini-Review. Exercise-induced 'browning' of adipose tissues. Metabolism 2018. Vol. 81, 63-70.
15. Cannon, B. & Nedergaard, J. Brown adipose tissue: function and physiological significance. Physiol. Rev 2004. 84, 277–359.
16. Whittle, A. Searching for ways to switch on brown fat: are we getting warmer? J. Mol. Endocrinol 2012. 49, R79–R87.
17. Lee, P. et al. Temperature-acclimated brown adipose tissue modulates insulin sensitivity in humans. Diabetes 2014. 63, 3686–3698.
18. Whittle, A., Relat-Pardo, J. & Vidal-Puig, A. Pharmacological strategies for targeting BAT thermogenesis. Trends Pharmacol. Sci. 2013. 34, 347–355.
19. Schwartz MW, Woods SC, Porte D Jr, Seeley RJ, Baskin DG. Central nervous system control of food intake. Nature 2000. 404:661–71.
20. Wanders, A. J., van den Borne, J. J. G. C., De Graaf, C., Hulshof, T., Jonathan, M. C., Kristensen, M., et al. Effects of dietary fibre on subjective appetite, energy intake and body weight: a systematic review of randomized controlled trials. Obesity Reviews 2011. 12(9), 724e739.
21. Caleigh M. Sawicki, Kara A. Livingston, Martin Obin, Susan B. Roberts, Mei Chung, and Nicola M. McKeown. Dietary Fiber and the Human Gut Microbiota: Application of Evidence Mapping Methodology. Nutrients. 2017 Feb; 9(2): 125.
22. Clark, M. J., & Slavin, J. L. The effect of fiber on satiety and food intake: a systematic review. Journal of the American College of Nutrition 2013. 32(3), 200e211.
23. Siri-Tarino PW, Sun Q, Hu FB, Krauss RM. Meta-analysis of prospective cohort studies evaluating the association of saturated fat with cardiovascular disease. Am J Clin Nutr. 2010. 91(3):535-46.
24. Barbara V. Howard; Linda Van Horn; Judith Hsia, MD; et al. Low-Fat Dietary Pattern and Risk of Cardiovascular Disease. The Women's Health Initiative Randomized Controlled Dietary Modification Trial. JAMA. 2006;295(6):655-666.

25. Mozaffarian, D., Pischon, T., Hankinson, S. E., Rifai, N., Joshipura, K., Willett, W. C. & Rimm, E. B. Dietary intake of trans fatty acids and systemic inflammation in women. Am. J. Clin. Nutr 2004. 79:606–612.
26. Gray B, Steyn F, Davies PS, Vitetta L. Omega-3 fatty acids: a review of the effects on adiponectin and leptin and potential implications for obesity management. Eur J Clin Nutr. 2013. 67(12):1234-42.
27. Sneddon AA, Tsofliou F, Fyfe CL, Matheson I, Jackson DM, Horgan G, Winzell MS, Wahle KW, Ahren B, Williams LM. Effect of a conjugated linoleic acid and omega-3 fatty acid mixture on body composition and adiponectin. Obesity (Silver Spring). 2008. 16(5):1019-24.
28. John C Kostyak, Penny Kris-Etherton, Deborah Bagshaw, James P DeLany and Peter A Farrell. Relative fat oxidation is higher in children than adults. Nutrition Journal 2007. 6:19.
29. Michael E.Holmstrup, Christopher M.Owens, Timothy J.Fairchild, Jill A.Kanaley. Effect of meal frequency on glucose and insulin excursions over the course of a day. e-SPEN, the European e-Journal of Clinical Nutrition and Metabolism 2010. Vol. 5, I6, 277-280.
30. Amy T. Hutchison, Leonie K. Heilbronn. Metabolic impacts of altering meal frequency and timing – Does when we eat matter? Biochimie 2016. Vol. 124, 187-197.
31. Accurso A, Bernstein RK, Dahlqvist A, et al. Dietary carbohydrate restriction in type 2 diabetes mellitus and metabolic syndrome : time for a critical appraisal. Nutr Metab 2008. 5 :9.
32. Valls-Pedret C, Sala-Vila A, Serr-Mir M, et al. Mediterranean diet and age-related cognitive decline : a randomised clinical trial. JAMA Intern Med. 2015.
33. Hartman AL, Lyle M, Rogawski MA, Gasior M. Efficacy of the ketogenic diet in the 6-hz seizure test. Epilepsia 2008. 49: 334–339.
34. Kessler SK, Neal EG, Camfield CS, Kossoff EH. Dietary therapies for epilepsy: future research. Epilepsy Behav 2011; 22: 17–22.
35. Warburg O. On respiratory impairment in cancer cells. Science 1956. 124: 269–270.
36. Pelicano H, Xu RH, Du M, Feng L, Sasaki R, Carew JS et al. Mitochondrial respiration defects in cancer cells cause activation of akt survival pathway through a redox-mediated mechanism. J Cell Biol 2006; 175: 913–923.
37. Ho VW, Leung K, Hsu A, Luk B, Lai J, Shen SY et al. A low carbohydrate, high protein diet slows tumor growth and prevents cancer initiation. Cancer Res 2011; 71: 4484–4493.
38. Seyfried BT, Kiebish M, Marsh J, Mukherjee P. Targeting energy metabolism in brain cancer through calorie restriction and the ketogenic diet. J Cancer Res Ther 2009; 5(Suppl 1): S7–S15.

39. A Paoli, A Rubini, JS Volek and KA Grimaldi. Beyond weight loss: a review of the therapeutic uses of very-low-carbohydrate (ketogenic) diets. European Journal of Clinical Nutrition 2013. 67, 789–796.
40. Johnstone AM, Horgan GW, Murison SD, Bremner DM, Lobley GE. Effects of a high-protein ketogenic diet on hunger, appetite, and weight loss in obese men feeding ad libitum. Am J Clin Nutr 2008. 87: 44–55.
41. Volek JS, Phinney SD, Forsythe CE, Quann EE, Wood RJ, Puglisi MJ et al. Carbohydrate restriction has a more favorable impact on the metabolic syndrome than a low fat diet. Lipids 2009. 44: 297–309.
42. Dashti HM, Al-Zaid NS, Mathew TC, Al-Mousawi M, Talib H, Asfar SK et al. Long term effects of ketogenic diet in obese subjects with high cholesterol level. Mol Cell Biochem 2006; 286: 1–9.
43. Yancy Jr WS, Foy M, Chalecki AM, Vernon MC, Westman EC. A low-carbohydrate, ketogenic diet to treat type 2 diabetes. Nutr Metab (Lond) 2005. 2: 34.
44. Westerterp-Plantenga MS, Nieuwenhuizen A, Tome D, Soenen S, Westerterp KR. Dietary protein, weight loss, and weight maintenance. Annu Rev Nutr 2009. 29: 21–41.
45. Leidy, H. J., Carnell, N. S., Mattes, R. D., & Campbell, W. W. Higher protein intake preserves lean mass and satiety with weight loss in pre-obese and obese women. Obesity 2007. 15(2), 421e429.
46. Paddon-Jones, D., Westman, E., Mattes, R. D., Wolfe, R. R., Astrup, A., & Westerterp-Plantenga, M. Protein, weight management, and satiety. American Journal of Clinical Nutrition 2008. 87(5), 1558Se1561S.
47. Weigle, D. S., Breen, P. A., Matthys, C. C., Callahan, H. S., Meeuws, K. E., Burden, V. R., et al. A high-protein diet induces sustained reductions in appetite, ad libitum caloric intake, and body weight despite compensatory changes in diurnal plasma leptin and ghrelin concentrations. American Journal of Clinical Nutrition 2005. 82(1), 41e48.
48. Westerterp-Plantenga, M., Lejeune, M., Nijs, I., Van Ooijen, M., & Kovacs, E. High protein intake sustains weight maintenance after body weight loss in humans. International Journal of Obesity 2004. 28(1), 57e64.
49. Metges CC, Barth CA. Metabolic consequences of a high dietary-protein intake in adulthood: assessment of the available evidence. J Nutr. 2000. 130:886–889.
50. William F Martin, Lawrence E Armstrong, and Nancy R Rodriguez. Dietary protein intake and renal function. Nutr Metab (Lond). 2005; 2: 25.
51. Havel PJ, Elliott SS, Tschoep M, et al. Consuming high fructose meals reduces 24 hour circulating insulin and leptin concentrations and does not suppress circulating ghrelin in women. J Invest Med 2002. 50:26A.

52. Cavadini C, Siega-Riz AM, Popkin BM. US adolescent food intake trends from 1965 to 1996. Arch Dis Child 2000. 83:18–24.
53. David S Ludwig, Karen E Peterson, Steven L Gortmaker. Relation between consumption of sugar-sweetened drinks and childhood obesity: a prospective, observational analysis. The Lancet 2001. Vol. 357, I9255, 505-508.
54. Poppitt SD, Keogh GF, Prentice AM, et al. Long-term effects of ad libitum low-fat, high-carbohydrate diets on body weight and serum lipids in overweight subjects with metabolic syndrome. Am J Clin Nutr 2002. 75:11–20.
55. Nordmann AJ, Nordmann A, Briel M, Keller U, Yancy Jr WS, Brehm BJ et al. Effects of low-carbohydrate vs low-fat diets on weight loss and cardiovascular risk factors: a meta-analysis of randomized controlled trials. Arch Intern Med 2006. 166: 285–293.
56. Shai I, Schwarzfuchs D, Henkin Y, Shahar DR, Witkow S, Greenberg I et al. Weight loss with a low-carbohydrate, mediterranean, or low-fat diet. N Engl J Med 2008. 359: 229–241.
57. Christina-Maria Kastorini, Haralampos J. Milionis, Katherine Esposito, Dario Giugliano, John A. Goudevenos, and Demosthenes B. Panagiotakos. The Effect of Mediterranean Diet on Metabolic Syndrome and its Components A Meta-Analysis of 50 Studies and 534,906 Individuals. J Am Coll Cardiol, 2011. 57:1299-1313
58. A Greenberg, James & Geliebter, Allan. Coffee, Hunger, and Peptide YY. Journal of the American College of Nutrition 2012. 31. 160-6.
59. Efthimia Karra, Keval Chandarana, and Rachel L Batterham. The role of peptide YY in appetite regulation and obesity. J Physiol. 2009. 587(Pt 1): 19–25.
60. Corney RA, Sunderland C, James LJ. Immediate pre-meal water ingestion decreases voluntary food intake in lean young males. Eur J Nutr. 2016. 55(2):815-819.
61. Muckelbauer R, Sarganas G, Grüneis A, Müller-Nordhorn J. Association between water consumption and body weight outcomes: a systematic review. Am J Clin Nutr. 2013. 98(2):282-99.
62. Ann C Skulas-Ray, Penny M Kris-Etherton, William S Harris, John P Vanden Heuvel, Paul R Wagner, Sheila G West. Dose-response effects of omega-3 fatty acids on triglycerides, inflammation, and endothelial function in healthy persons with moderate hypertriglyceridemia. The American Journal of Clinical Nutrition 2011. Vol. 93, I2, 243–252.
63. Frauchiger MT, Wenk C, Colombani PC. Effects of acute chromium supplementation on postprandial metabolism in healthy young men. J Am Coll Nutr. 2004. 23(4):351-7.3.
64. Quann, EE, Silvestre R, Kirwan JP, Sharman MJ, Judelson DA, Spiering BA, Vingren JL, Maresh CM, VanHeest JL, Kraemer WJ, Volek JS.

Effects of chromium supplementation on glycogen synthesis and insulin signaling after high-intensity exercise. Am Coll Sports Med. 2006. 10.
65. Mason C, Xiao L, Imayama I, Duggan C, Wang CY, Korde L, McTiernan A. Vitamin D3 supplementation during weight loss: a double-blind randomized controlled trial. Am J Clin Nutr. 2014. 99(5):1015-25.
66. Salehpour A, Hosseinpanah F, Shidfar F, Vafa M, Razaghi M, Dehghani S, Hoshiarrad A, Gohari M. A 12-week double-blind randomized clinical trial of vitamin D_3 supplementation on body fat mass in healthy overweight and obese women. Nutr J. 2012. 22;11:78.
67. Parikh SJ, Edelman M, Uwaifo GI, Freedman RJ, Semega-Janneh M, Reynolds J, Yanovski JA. The relationship between obesity and serum 1,25-dihydroxy vitamin D concentrations in healthy adults. J Clin Endocrinol Metab. 2004. 89(3):1196-9.
68. Klaus W.Lange, JoachimHauser, Yukiko Nakamura, Shigehiko Kanaya. Dietary seaweeds and obesity. Food Science and Human Wellness 2015. Vol. 4, I3, 87-96.
69. Min Sun Kim, Jung Yun Kim, Woong Hwan Choi, and Sang Sun Lee. Effects of seaweed supplementation on blood glucose concentration, lipid profile, and antioxidant enzyme activities in patients with type 2 diabetes mellitus. Nutr Res Pract. 2008. 2(2): 62–67.
70. Yi Ding, YuWen Li, AiDong Wen. Effect of niacin on lipids and glucose in patients with type 2 diabetes: A meta-analysis of randomized, controlled clinical trials. Clinical Nutrition 2015. Vol. 34, I5, 838-844.
71. Chen HY, Cheng FC, Pan HC, Hsu JC, Wang MF. Magnesium enhances exercise performance via increasing glucose availability in the blood, muscle, and brain during exercise. PLoS One. 2014. 20;9(1):e85486.
72. Veronese N, Berton L, Carraro S, Bolzetta F, De Rui M, Perissinotto E, Toffanello ED, Bano G, Pizzato S, Miotto F, Coin A, Manzato E, Sergi G. Effect of oral magnesium supplementation on physical performance in healthy elderly women involved in a weekly exercise program: a randomized controlled trial. Am J Clin Nutr. 2014. 100(3):974-81.
73. Setaro L, Santos-Silva PR, Nakano EY, Sales CH, Nunes N, Greve JM, Colli C. Magnesium status and the physical performance of volleyball players: effects of magnesium supplementation. J Sports Sci. 2014;32(5):438-45.
74. Barragán-Rodríguez L, Rodríguez-Morán M, Guerrero-Romero F. Efficacy and safety of oral magnesium supplementation in the treatment of depression in the elderly with type 2 diabetes: a randomized, equivalent trial. Magnes Res. 2008. 21(4):218-23.
75. Kim DJ, Xun P, Liu K, Loria C, Yokota K, Jacobs DR Jr, He K. Magnesium intake in relation to systemic inflammation, insulin resistance, and the incidence of diabetes. Diabetes Care. 2010. 33(12):2604-10.

76. Chacko SA, Sul J, Song Y, Li X, LeBlanc J, You Y, Butch A, Liu S. Magnesium supplementation, metabolic and inflammatory markers, and global genomic and proteomic profiling: a randomized, double-blind, controlled, crossover trial in overweight individuals. Am J Clin Nutr. 2011. 93(2):463-73.
77. Mooren FC, Krüger K, Völker K, Golf SW, Wadepuhl M, Kraus A. Oral magnesium supplementation reduces insulin resistance in non-diabetic subjects - a double-blind, placebo-controlled, randomized trial. Diabetes Obes Metab. 2011. 13(3):281-4.
78. Leslie M.Klevay. Is the Western diet adequate in copper? Journal of Trace Elements in Medicine and Biology 2011. Vol. 25, I4, 204-212.
79. Garrido-Maraver J, Cordero MD, Oropesa-Avila M, Vega AF, de la Mata M, Pavon AD, Alcocer-Gomez E, Calero CP, Paz MV, Alanis M, de Lavera I, Cotan D, Sanchez-Alcazar JA. Clinical applications of coenzyme Q10. Front Biosci (Landmark Ed). 2014. 19:619-33.
80. Amin MM, Asaad GF, Abdel Salam RM, El-Abhar HS, Arbid MS. Novel CoQ10 antidiabetic mechanisms underlie its positive effect: modulation of insulin and adiponectine receptors, Tyrosine kinase, PI3K, glucose transporters, sRAGE and visfatin in insulin resistant/diabetic rats. PLoS One. 2014. 20;9(2):e89169.
81. Kent Sahlin. Boosting fat burning with carnitine: an old friend comes out from the shadow. J Physiol. 2011. 589(Pt 7): 1509–1510.
82. Francis B Stephens, Dumitru Constantin-Teodosiu, and Paul L Greenhaff. New insights concerning the role of carnitine in the regulation of fuel metabolism in skeletal muscle. J Physiol. 2007. 581(Pt 2): 431–444.
83. Rosca MG, Lemieux H, Hoppel CL. Mitochondria in the elderly: Is acetylcarnitine a rejuvenator? Adv Drug Deliv Rev. 2009. 30;61(14):1332-1342.
84. Pooyandjoo M, Nouhi M, Shab-Bidar S, Djafarian K, Olyaeemanesh A. The effect of (L-)carnitine on weight loss in adults: a systematic review and meta-analysis of randomized controlled trials. Obes Rev. 2016. 17(10):970-6.
85. Kraemer WJ, Volek JS, French DN, Rubin MR, Sharman MJ, Gómez AL, Ratamess NA, Newton RU, Jemiolo B, Craig BW, Häkkinen K. The effects of L-carnitine L-tartrate supplementation on hormonal responses to resistance exercise and recovery. J Strength Cond Res. 2003. 17(3):455-62.
86. Kulkarni, S.K., Bhutani, M.K. & Bishnoi, M. Antidepressant activity of curcumin: involvement of serotonin and dopamine system. Psychopharmacology 2008. 201: 435.
87. Bharat B. Aggarwal, Kuzhuvelil B. Harikumar. Potential therapeutic effects of curcumin, the anti-inflammatory agent, against neurodegenerative, cardiovascular, pulmonary, metabolic, autoimmune

and neoplastic diseases. The International Journal of Biochemistry & Cell Biology 2009. Vol. 41, I1, 40-59.
88. Biswas SK, McClure D, Jimenez LA, Megson IL, Rahman I. Curcumin induces glutathione biosynthesis and inhibits NF-kappaB activation and interleukin-8 release in alveolar epithelial cells: mechanism of free radical scavenging activity. Antioxid Redox Signal. 2005. 7(1-2):32-41.
89. Carey N. Lumeng and Alan R. Saltiel. Inflammatory links between obesity and metabolic disease. J Clin Invest. 2011. 121(6):2111–2117.
90. Shao W, Yu Z, Chiang Y, Yang Y, Chai T, Foltz W, Lu H, Fantus IG, Jin T. Curcumin prevents high fat diet induced insulin resistance and obesity via attenuating lipogenesis in liver and inflammatory pathway in adipocytes. PLoS ONE. 2012. 7:e28784.17.
91. Judith L Ngondi, Julius E Oben, and Samuel R Minka. The effect of Irvingia gabonensis seeds on body weight and blood lipids of obese subjects in Cameroon. Lipids Health Dis. 2005; 4: 12.
92. Oben JE, Ngondi JL, Momo CN, Agbor GA, Sobgui CS. The use of a Cissus quadrangularis/Irvingia gabonensis combination in the management of weight loss: a double-blind placebo-controlled study. Lipids Health Dis. 2008. 7:12.
93. Ngondi JL, Etoundi BC, Nyangono CB, Mbofung CM, Oben JE. IGOB131, a novel seed extract of the West African plant Irvingia gabonensis, significantly reduces body weight and improves metabolic parameters in overweight humans in a randomized double-blind placebo controlled investigation. Lipids Health Dis. 2009. 2;8:7.
94. Ross SM. African mango (IGOB131): a proprietary seed extract of Irvingia gabonensis is found to be effective in reducing body weight and improving metabolic parameters in overweight humans. Holist Nurs Pract. 2011. 25(4):215-7.
95. Venables MC, Hulston CJ, Cox HR, Jeukendrup AE. Green tea extract ingestion, fat oxidation, and glucose tolerance in healthy humans. Am J Clin Nutr. 2008. 87(3):778-84.
96. AG Dulloo, J Seydoux, L Girardier, P Chantre & J Vandermander. Green tea and thermogenesis: interactions between catechin-polyphenols, caffeine and sympathetic activity. International Journal of Obesity 2000. Vol. 24, 252–258.
97. M.S.Westerterp-Plantenga. Green tea catechins, caffeine and body-weight regulation. Physiology & Behavior 2010. Vol. 100, I1, 42-46.
98. Yun JM, Jialal I, Devaraj S. Effects of epigallocatechin gallate on regulatory T cell number and function in obese v. lean volunteers. Br J Nutr. 2010. 103:1771–7.18.
99. Liu K, Zhou R, Wang B, Mi MT. Effect of resveratrol on glucose control and insulin sensitivity: a meta-analysis of 11 randomized controlled trials. Am J Clin Nutr. 2014. 99(6):1510-9.

100. Kuršvietienė L, Stanevičienė I, Mongirdienė A, Bernatonienė J. Multiplicity of effects and health benefits of resveratrol. Medicina (Kaunas). 2016. 52(3):148-55.
101. Lee JH, Moon MH, Jeong JK, Park YG, Lee YJ, Seol JW, Park SY. Sulforaphane induced adipolysis via hormone sensitive lipase activation, regulated by AMPK signaling pathway. Biochem Biophys Res Commun. 2012. 426(4):492-7.
102. Vomhof-Dekrey EE, Picklo MJ Sr. The Nrf2-antioxidant response element pathway: a target for regulating energy metabolism. J Nutr Biochem 2012. 23(10):1201-6.
103. Choi KM, Lee YS, Sin DM, Lee S, Lee MK, Lee YM, Hong JT, Yun YP, Yoo HS. Sulforaphane inhibits mitotic clonal expansion during adipogenesis through cell cycle arrest. Obesity (Silver Spring). 2012. 20: 1365–71.
104. Slavin J. Fiber and prebiotics: mechanisms and health benefits. Nutrients. 2013. 22;5(4):1417-35.
105. Mattia P. Arena, Graziano Caggianiello, Daniela Fiocco, Pasquale Russo, Michele Torelli, Giuseppe Spano, and Vittorio Capozzi. Barley β-Glucans-Containing Food Enhances Probiotic Performances of Beneficial Bacteria. Int J Mol Sci. 2014. 15(2): 3025–3039.

Chapter Four – Metabolism

1. James Groff, Sareen Gropper. Advanced Nutrition and Human Metabolism. Wadsworth 2000.
2. Martin Kohlmeier. Nutrient Metabolism. Academic Press 2015.
3. Bouché C, Serdy S, Kahn C, Goldfine A. The cellular fate of glucose and its relevance in type 2 diabetes. Endocr Rev. 2004. 25 (5): 807–30.
4. Demirel Y, Sandler S. Thermodynamics and bioenergetics. Biophys Chem 2002. 97 (2–3): 87–111.
5. Brand M. Regulation analysis of energy metabolism. J Exp Biol 1997. 200 (Pt 2): 193–202.
6. Stiegler P, Cunliffe A. The role of diet and exercise for the maintenance of fat-free mass and resting metabolic rate during weight loss. Sports Medicine 2006. 36 (3): 239–262.
7. Johnstone AM, Murison SD, Duncan JS, Rance KA, Speakman JR, Koh YO. Factors influencing variation in basal metabolic rate include fat-free mass, fat mass, age, and circulating thyroxine but not sex, circulating leptin, or triiodothyronine. American Journal of Clinical Nutrition 2005. 82 (5): 941–948.
8. Speakman JR, Król E, Johnson MS. The Functional Significance of Individual Variation in Basal Metabolic Rate. Physiological and Biochemical Zoology 2004. 77 (6): 900–915.

9. Broeder, CE; Burrhus, KA; Svanevik, LS; Wilmore, JH. The effects of aerobic fitness on resting metabolic rate. The American Journal of Clinical Nutrition 1992. 55 (4): 795–801.
10. Pratley, R; Nicklas, B; Rubin, M; Miller, J; Smith, A; Smith, M; Hurley, B; Goldberg, A. Strength training increases resting metabolic rate and norepinephrine levels in healthy 50- to 65-year-old men. Journal of Applied Physiology 1994. 76 (1): 133–137.
11. Grattan BJ Jr; Connolly-Schoonen J. Addressing weight loss recidivism: a clinical focus on metabolic rate and the psychological aspects of obesity. ISRN Obesity. 2012: 567530.
12. Tsai, AG; Wadden, TA. Systematic review: An evaluation of major commercial weight loss programs in the United States. Annals of Internal Medicine 2005. 142 (1): 56–66.
13. Thompson D, Karpe F, Lafontan M, Frayn K. Physical activity and exercise in the regulation of human adipose tissue physiology. Physiol Rev. 2012 Jan;92(1):157-91.
14. Carla E. Cox. Role of Physical Activity for Weight Loss and Weight Maintenance. Diabetes Spectrum 2017. 30(3): 157-160.
15. Polak J, Klimcakova E, Moro C, Viguerie N, Berlan M, Hejnova J, Richterova B, Kraus I, Langin D, Stich V. Effect of aerobic training on plasma levels and subcutaneous abdominal adipose tissue gene expression of adiponectin, leptin, interleukin 6, and tumor necrosis factor alpha in obese women. Metabolism. 2006 Oct;55(10):1375-81.
16. Mikines KJ, Sonne B, Farrell PA, Tronier B, Galbo H. Effect of training on the dose-response relationship for insulin action in men. J Appl Physiol 1985. 66(2):695-703.
17. Schulz LO, Nyomba BL, Alger S, Anderson TE, Ravussin E. Effect of endurance training on sedentary energy expenditure measured in a respiratory chamber. Am J Physiol. 1991. Feb; 260(2 Pt 1):E257-61.
18. Jeffrey E. Herrick, Gino S. Panza, and Jared M. Gollie. Leptin, Leptin Soluble Receptor, and the Free Leptin Index following a Diet and Physical Activity Lifestyle Intervention in Obese Males and Females. Journal of Obesity 2016. Art. ID 8375828, 5 pages.
19. Siham Yasari, Donghao Wang, Denis Prud'homme, Marek Jankowski, Jolanta Gutkowska, Jean-Marc Lavoie. Exercise training decreases plasma leptin levels and the expression of hepatic leptin receptor-a, -b, and, -e in rats. Molecular and Cellular Biochemistry 2009. 324:13.
20. Javier T. Gonzalez, Rachel C. Veasey, Penny L. S. Rumbold, Emma J. Stevenson. Breakfast and exercise contingently affect postprandial metabolism and energy balance in physically active males. British Journal of Nutrition, 2013; 1.

21. Wilmore J.; Knuttgen H. Aerobic Exercise and Endurance Improving Fitness for Health Benefits. The Physician and Sportsmedicine 2003. 31 (5): 45.
22. De Vos N.; Singh N.; Ross D.; Stavrinos T. Optimal Load for Increasing Muscle Power During Explosive Resistance Training in Older Adults. The Journals of Gerontology 2005. 60A (5): 638–647.
23. Egan B, Zierath JR. Exercise metabolism and the molecular regulation of skeletal muscle adaptation. Cell Metabolism 2013. 17 (2): 162–184.
24. Lee, I-Min; Shiroma, Eric J; Lobelo, Felipe; Puska, Pekka; Blair, Steven N; Katzmarzyk, Peter T. Impact of Physical Inactivity on the World's Major Non-Communicable Diseases. Lancet 2012. 380 (9838): 219–229.
25. Milanović, Z; Sporiš, G; Weston, M. Effectiveness of High-Intensity Interval Training (HIT) and Continuous Endurance Training for VO2max Improvements: A Systematic Review and Meta-Analysis of Controlled Trials. Sports Medicine 2015. 45 (10): 1469–81.
26. Swardfager W. Exercise intervention and inflammatory markers in coronary artery disease: a meta-analysis. Am. Heart J 2012. 163 (4): 666–76.
27. Denham J, Marques FZ, O'Brien BJ, Charchar FJ. Exercise: putting action into our epigenome. Sports Med 2104. 44 (2): 189–209.
28. Erickson KI, Miller DL, Roecklein KA. The aging hippocampus: interactions between exercise, depression, and BDNF. Neuroscientist 2012. 18 (1): 82–97.
29. Basso JC, Suzuki WA. The Effects of Acute Exercise on Mood, Cognition, Neurophysiology, and Neurochemical Pathways: A Review. Brain Plasticity 2017. 2 (2): 127–152.
30. Halton, T. L., & Hu, F. B. The effects of high protein diets on thermogenesis, satiety and weight loss: a critical review. Journal of the American College of Nutrition 2004, 23(5), 373e385.
31. Peter Aldiss, James Betts, Craig Sale, Mark Pope, Helen Budge, Michael E. Symonds. Mini-Review. Exercise-induced 'browning' of adipose tissues. Metabolism 2018. Vol. 81, 63-70.
32. Westerterp-Plantenga, M., Rolland, V., Wilson, S., & Westerterp, K. Satiety related to 24 h diet-induced thermogenesis during high protein/carbohydrate vs high fat diets measured in a respiration chamber. European Journal of Clinical Nutrition 1999. 53(6), 495e502.
33. Bostrom, P. et al. A PGC1-alpha-dependent myokine that drives brown-fat-like development of white fat and thermogenesis. Nature 2012. 481, 463–468.
34. Cypess, A. M. et al. Identification and importance of brown adipose tissue in adult humans. N. Engl. J. Med 2009. 360, 1509–1517.

35. Nedergaard, J., Bengtsson, T. & Cannon, B. Unexpected evidence for active brown adipose tissue in adult humans. Am. J. Physiol. Endocrinol. Metab 2007. 293, E444–E452.
36. Ouellet, V. et al. Outdoor temperature, age, sex, body mass index, and diabetic status determine the prevalence, mass, and glucose-uptake activity of 18F-FDG-detected BAT in humans. J. Clin. Endocrinol. Metab 2011. 96, 192–199.
37. Cannon, B. & Nedergaard, J. Brown adipose tissue: function and physiological significance. Physiol. Rev 2004. 84, 277–359.
38. Whittle, A. Searching for ways to switch on brown fat: are we getting warmer? J. Mol. Endocrinol 2012. 49, R79–R87.
39. Lee, P. et al. Temperature-acclimated brown adipose tissue modulates insulin sensitivity in humans. Diabetes 2014. 63, 3686–3698.
40. Bartelt, A. et al. Brown adipose tissue activity controls triglyceride clearance. Nat. Med 2011. 17, 200–205.
41. Whittle, A. J. et al. Soluble LR11/SorLA represses thermogenesis in adipose tissue and correlates with BMI in humans. Nat. Commun 2015. 6:8951.
42. Schulz, T. J. et al. Brown-fat paucity due to impaired BMP signalling induces compensatory browning of white fat. Nature 2013. 495, 379–383.
43. Schulz, T. J. et al. Identification of inducible brown adipocyte progenitors residing in skeletal muscle and white fat. Proc. Natl Acad. Sci. USA 2011. 108, 143–148.
44. Klinger, S. C. et al. SorLA regulates the activity of lipoprotein lipase by intracellular trafficking. J. Cell. Sci. 2011. 124, 1095–1105.
45. Whittle, A., Relat-Pardo, J. & Vidal-Puig, A. Pharmacological strategies for targeting BAT thermogenesis. Trends Pharmacol. Sci. 2013. 34, 347–355.
46. Jéquier E, Tappy L. Regulation of body weight in humans. Physiol Rev 1999. 79:451–80.
47. Romieu I, Willett WC, Stampfer MJ, et al. Energy intake and other determinants of relative weight. Am J Clin Nutr 1988. 47:406–12.
48. Feskens EJ, Virtanen SM, Rasanen L, et al. Dietary factors determining diabetes and impaired glucose tolerance. A 20-year follow-up of the Finnish and Dutch cohorts of the Seven Countries Study. Diabetes Care 1995. 18:1104–12.
49. Weigle DS, Duell PB, Connor WE, Steiner RA, Soules MR, Kuijper JL. Effect of fasting, refeeding, and dietary fat restriction on plasma leptin levels. J Clin Endocrinol Metab 1997. 82:561–5.
50. Jelleyman C, Yates T, O'Donovan G, Gray LJ, King JA, Khunti K, Davies MJ (November 2015). "The effects of high-intensity interval training on glucose regulation and insulin resistance: a meta-analysis". Obes Rev (Meta-Analysis). 16 (11): 942–61. doi:10.1111/obr.12317.

51. Trapp, E. G.; Chisholm, D. J.; Freund, J.; Boutcher, S. H. (2008-01-15). "The effects of high-intensity intermittent exercise training on fat loss and fasting insulin levels of young women". International Journal of Obesity. 32 (4): 684–691. doi:10.1038/sj.ijo.0803781.
52. Talanian, Jason L.; Galloway, Stuart D. R.; Heigenhauser, George J. F.; Bonen, Arend; Spriet, Lawrence L. (April 2007). "Two weeks of high-intensity aerobic interval training increases the capacity for fat oxidation during exercise in women". Journal of Applied Physiology. 102 (4): 1439–1447. doi:10.1152/japplphysiol.01098.2006.
53. Boutcher, Stephen H. (2011). "High-Intensity Intermittent Exercise and Fat Loss". Journal of Obesity. 2011: 868305. doi:10.1155/2011/868305.
54. Tabata, Izumi; Nishimura, Kouji; Kouzaki, Motoki; Hirai, Yuusuke; Ogita, Futoshi; Miyachi, Motohiko; Yamamoto, Kaoru (1996). "Effects of moderate-intensity endurance and high-intensity intermittent training on anaerobic capacity and VO2max" (PDF). Medicine & Science in Sports & Exercise. 28 (10): 1327–1330.
55. Tabata, Izumi; Irisawa, Kouichi; Kouzaki, Motoki; Nishimura, Kouji; Ogita, Futoshi; Miyachi, Motohiko (1997). "Metabolic profile of high intensity intermittent exercises". Medicine & Science in Sports & Exercise. 29 (3): 390–5.
56. Francisco Acosta et al. Physiological responses to acute cold exposure in young lean men PLoS One. 2018; 13(5): e0196543.
57. Yann Ravussin, Cuiying Xiao, Oksana Gavrilova and Marc L. Reitman, Effect of Intermittent Cold Exposure on Brown Fat Activation, Obesity, and Energy Homeostasis in Mice, PLoS One. 2014; 9(1): e85876.
58. Presby DM, Jackman MR, Rudolph MC, Sherk VD, Foright RM, Houck JA, Johnson GC, Orlicky DJ, Melanson EL, Higgins JA, MacLean PS. Compensation for cold-induced thermogenesis during weight loss maintenance and regain. Am J Physiol Endocrinol Metab. 2019 May 1;316(5):E977-E986.
59. Marlatt KL, Ravussin E. Brown Adipose Tissue: an Update on Recent Findings. Curr Obes Rep. 2017 Dec;6(4):389-396.
60. Poekes L, Lanthier N, Leclercq IA. Brown adipose tissue: a potential target in the fight against obesity and the metabolic syndrome. Clin Sci (Lond). 2015 Dec;129(11):933-49.

DISCLAIMER

The information in this book is not intended or implied to be a substitute for professional medical advice, diagnosis or treatment. All content, including text, graphics, images and information, contained in or available through this book is for general information purposes only. Whenever commencing a weight-loss programme always consult with your doctor or medical practitioner first.

Printed in Great Britain
by Amazon